Department of Veterans Affairs
Health Services Research & Development Service

Evidence-based Synthesis Program

Strategies for Suicide Prevention in Veterans

January 2009

Prepared for:

Department of Veterans Affairs
Veterans Health Administration
Health Services Research & Development Service
Washington, DC 20420

Prepared by:

Greater Los Angeles Veterans Affairs Healthcare
System/Southern California/RAND Evidence-based
Practice Center
Los Angeles, CA

Investigators

Paul Shekelle, MD, PhD
Director

Steven Bagley, MD, MS
Content Expert/Physician Reviewer

Brett Munjas, BA
Project Manager/Literature Database Manager

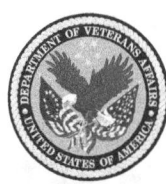

PREFACE

VA's Health Services Research and Development Service (HSR&D) works to improve the cost, quality, and outcomes of health care for our nation's veterans. Collaborating with VA leaders, managers, and policy makers, HSR&D focuses on important health care topics that are likely to have significant impact on quality improvement efforts. One significant collaborative effort is HSR&D's Evidence-based Synthesis Pilot Project (ESP). Through this project, HSR&D provides timely and accurate evidence syntheses on targeted health care topics. These products will be disseminated broadly throughout VA and will: inform VA clinical policy, develop clinical practice guidelines, set directions for future research to address gaps in knowledge, identify the evidence to support VA performance measures, and rationalize drug formulary decisions.

HSR&D provided funding for the two Evidence Based Practice Centers (EPCs) supported by the Agency for Healthcare Research and Quality (AHRQ) that also had an active and publicly acknowledged VA affiliation—Southern California EPC and Portland, OR EPC—so they could develop evidence syntheses on requested topics for dissemination to VA policymakers. A planning committee with representation from HSR&D, Patient Care Services, Office of Quality and Performance, and the VISN Clinical Management Officers, has been established to identify priority topics and to insure the quality of final reports.

Comments on this evidence report are welcome and can be sent to Susan Schiffner, ESP Program Manager, at Susan.Schiffner@va.gov.

TABLE OF CONTENTS

STRATEGIES FOR SUICIDE PREVENTION IN VETERANS

EXECUTIVE SUMMARY

BACKGROUND

Suicide is a devastating outcome of major public health importance. Suicide rates for patients abusing alcohol and other substances, or suffering from other mental health conditions may be elevated. Because suicide prevention is a priority of the Veterans Health Administration, the VA wishes to expand and enhance use of evidence-based prevention or reduction methods..

The Key Questions were:

Key Question 1. What are the new or improved suicide prevention strategies (e.g. hotlines, outreach programs, peer counseling, treatment coordination programs, and new counseling approaches) that show promise for Veterans?

Key Question 2. What solid evidence base supports the most promising strategies?

Key Question 3. What evidence is still needed to establish various strategies as the most promising (framed as research questions to guide and focus continued research to expand knowledge regarding the effectiveness of suicide prevention approaches)?

METHODS
Mann et al. completed a systematic review of the literature on suicide prevention from 1966 through June 2005.[1] They searched MEDLINE, the Cochrane Library, and PsychINFO databases. We updated this using the same search strategy, starting from June 2005 through May 2008. Only studies reporting direct effects of interventions on suicide attempts or completions were considered. Studies reporting results from any country for military or veterans were included, as were studies in Anglo/American countries with adult populations reporting interventions other than strictly mental-health interventions. Titles, abstracts, and articles were reviewed by a psychiatrist trained in the critical analysis of literature. Data were narratively summarized.

RESULTS
We screened 3,406 titles and performed a more detailed review on 261 articles. We identified seven multifaceted studies of military personnel, five in the US, and two multifaceted national suicide prevention programs. We identified three studies of US veterans. We found 20 randomized or controlled clinical trials of interventions post-suicide attempt. We found a large number of observational studies of restricting access to lethal means, and a small number of heterogeneous trials and studies.

KEY QUESTION #1: What are the new or improved suicide prevention strategies (e.g. hotlines, outreach programs, peer counseling, treatment coordination programs, and new counseling approaches) that show promise for Veterans?

KEY QUESTION #2: What solid evidence base supports the most promising strategies?
Multicomponent interventions in military personnel probably reduce the risk of suicide. The largest and best described such study was implemented for the US Air Force, and this study provides the most convincing evidence of effectiveness. The report of success of a program in Yugoslavia modeled after the USAF program increases our confidence that the effect is real. A similar program was developed for the US Navy and Marine Corps. However, as with any multicomponent intervention shown to be successful, there are still numerous questions about the relative merit of inclusion of each individual component (could the same effect be achieved with fewer components?) or the possible increase in effectiveness of adding other components, and optimizing the effectiveness of each additional component. Additionally, there are no data about its effect in non-military populations, although veterans would seem to be sufficiently close to a military population that some transferability of results could be assumed. (GRADE quality of evidence = Low, meaning further research is very likely to have an important impact on our confidence in the estimate of effect and is likely to change the estimate)

There are insufficient studies of suicide prevention programs specifically in veterans to draw conclusions (GRADE quality of evidence = Very Low, meaning any estimate of effect is uncertain)

Psychosocial interventions following a suicide attempt are, at the very best, only minimally effective (GRADE quality of evidence = Moderate, meaning further research is likely to have an important impact on our confidence in the estimate of the effect and may change the estimate).

There are insufficient data to reach conclusions about Community-based Suicide Prevention Centers (GRADE quality of evidence = Very Low , meaning any estimate of effect is uncertain)

We found no studies that assessed the specific effectiveness of any of hotlines, outreach programs as primary prevention interventions, peer counseling, treatment coordination programs, and new counseling programs.

Restriction of access to lethal means probably has an effect on cause-specific suicides, although its effect on total suicides is less clear (GRADE quality of evidence = Low, meaning further research is very likely to have an important impact on our confidence in the estimate of effect and is likely to change the estimate)

KEY QUESTION #3: What evidence is still needed to establish various strategies as the most promising (framed as research questions to guide and focus continued research to expand knowledge regarding the effectiveness of suicide prevention approaches)?

Multifaceted interventions are supported by consistent evidence, although of very mixed quality.

Even if such programs are later determined to be robustly successful, the question of which components in those programs are causally related to the reduction in suicides has not been addressed. This sets as a research issue determining which components work best in which combinations for which populations. The issue of whether some sets of components may have facilitative or synergistic effects has not been addressed.

Psychosocial intervention for suicide attempters have considerable face validity as they address a group with manifest evidence of suicide risk, but there is no consistent evidence in their support in spite of a moderate number of randomized controlled trials that been conducted. This is an area of obvious and considerable interest to the VA, which is now using similar approaches in its clinical programs to identify and track those at high risk with suicide risk flags, screening tools, and suicide prevention coordinators. An additional factor that seems relevant but rarely directly studied is the effect of forming a consistent relationship with a single provider, a therapeutic alliance, and its role in providing a protective degree of social connection, and reducing the harmful consequences of social isolation.

Further randomized controlled trials and high-quality observational studies are definitely needed. Without waiting for such to be completed, and independent of which program components the VA decides to pursue, there are two supporting initiatives that could be implemented in parallel. The first concerns standardizing vocabulary, and the second concerns electronic medical records.

First, all suicide prevention programs are dependent on the accuracy with which assessments of suicidality are conducted. The term "suicide attempt" covers a very broad array of self-injurious behaviors, from intentionally planned, high lethality events that were interrupted by mere happenstance, through low lethality acts marked by a small risk of physical harm, impulsivity, and a high likelihood of discovery by others. Others have noted the importance of establishing and using a consistent nomenclature in this area. It is critical for further advances in suicide reduction that such attempts are carried through.

A very important reason for accurately describing the severity of suicide attempts is that an attempt is widely recognized as a significant risk factor for completions. Although most completed suicides are first attempts[2] and attempters vary in important ways from completers,[3] it is known that survivors of highly lethal attempts have similar clinical and psychosocial profiles to antemorten profiles of suicide completers. This suggests that subcategorization of attempt by lethality (or perhaps other factors) may be clinically useful.

Second, because the VA uses a single, integrated computerized medical record system for all of its clinical activities, any improvements in vocabulary along with new screening and tracking tools would allow for data gathering as part of routine practice – especially for establishing patterns and risk factors for suicide attempts – in advance of formally conducted observational studies or controlled trials.

INTRODUCTION

BACKGROUND

Suicide is a major problem in public health. In the US suicide is roughly the 10th leading cause of death, corresponding to about 30,000 deaths per year. Suicide is now understood as a multifactorial phenomenon, with biological, psychological, and social/environmental risk vulnerabilities and triggers. The majority of suicides – at least 90% by some studies – in the US implicate a psychiatric disorder, usually a mood disorder.[1,2]

US military veterans are a large population with multiple, and often significant risk factors for suicide. The Veterans Health Study, which screened 2160 male outpatients at Boston-area VA clinics, reported depressive symptoms in 31% of the sample, a rate more than twice that of the general population.[4] A study of over 800,000 depressed veterans reported a suicide rate about 7 times higher than the baseline risk in the general population.[5] The same study also showed that substance abuse elevated the suicide risk in depressed veterans. A recent report on the prevalence of mental health disorders in soldiers returning from the current Iraq conflict found clinician-identified mental health problems in 20% of active duty personnel, and in over 40% of National Guard and reserve personnel.[6] Suicide in these newly discharged veterans has also received considerable political and media scrutiny.

The main problem confronting those working in suicide prevention is that while the absolute number of suicides in a population is cumulatively quite large, the risk of suicide to any given individual, even those with multiple risk factors, is by relative measures quite small. This problem is illustrated in an example in Gaynes et al.[7] who show that for reasonable assumptions of sensitivity and specificity, a screening test for suicide risk would have a positive predictive value of 0.3% and generate an overwhelming number of false positives. These same factors complicate any attempt at constructing randomized clinical trials of suicide prevention efforts. It is widely recognized that the problem of accurate suicide prediction at the clinical level is currently an intractable one.[3]

In spite of the difficulties with prediction, structured approaches to suicide prevention have been developed. The multifactorial nature of the problem of suicide has required the adoption of a multifaceted approach to intervention, combining population-based screening and education, with more targeted efforts for those at above-baseline risk. These methods were reviewed by Mann et al.[1] and their conceptual model will organize the interventions we review in this report (Figure 1).

Figure 1. Targets of Suicide Prevention Interventions from Mann et al.[1]

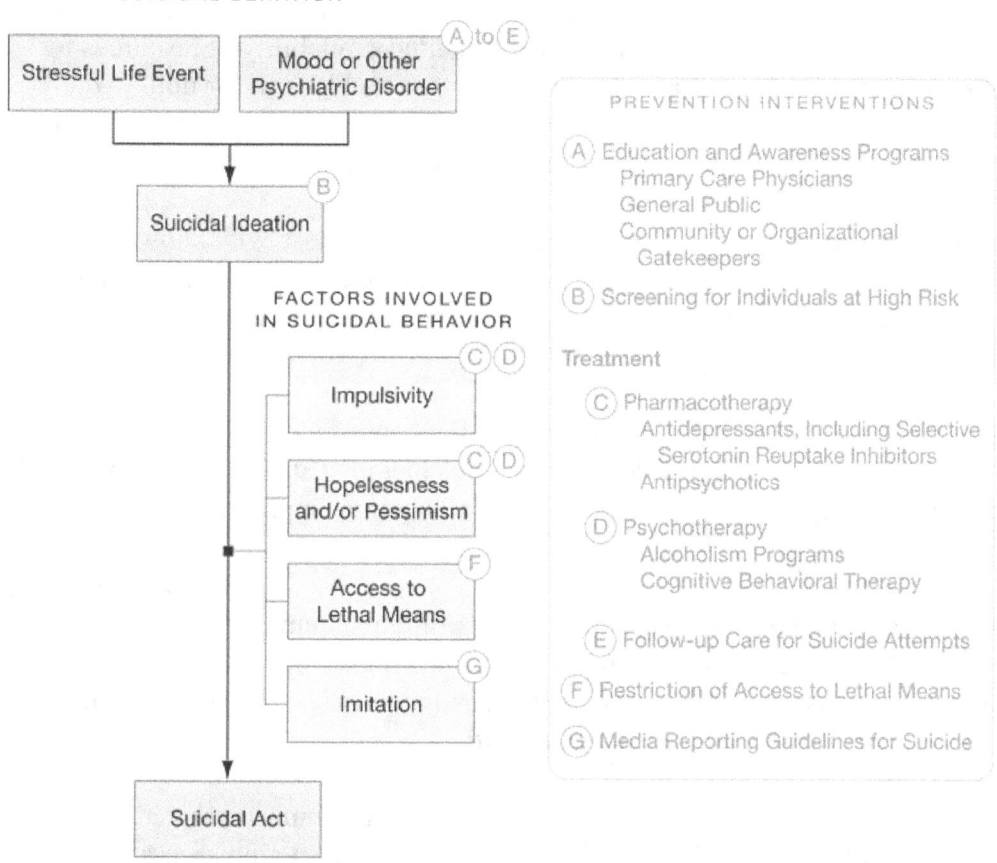

In their model life stressors and psychiatric disorders combine to produce suicidal ideation, which is modulated by impulsivity, hopelessness/pessimism, access to lethal means, and imitation, leading to the final suicidal act. The interventions correspond to different points in this causal network. The set of interventions, adapted from Mann et al., that are considered in this review appear in Table 1 and described in detail in the following.

Table 1. Set of interventions from Mann et al.[1]

Education and Awareness Programs
Primary Care Physicians
General Public/Population
Community or Organization Gatekeepers
Screening for individuals at high risk
Pharmacotherapy or ECT
Psychotherapy
Follow-up care for suicide attempts
Restriction of access to lethal means
Media reporting guidelines for suicide

Other Education and awareness programs can have various audiences; they can be aimed at primary care physicians to improve detection of mental health issues or significant stressors with the goal of referring to mental health clinicians for diagnosis and treatment, at a particular population (or the general public) to educate them about suicide and the availability of resources for getting help, and at nonclincian gatekeepers, such as medical clerks, chaplains, or military unit commanders, who as part of their work activities come into contact with large groups and who could, with improved training, provide education or identify those at high risk.

Screening programs for those at high risk target interventions towards those with known risk factors for suicide. These include patients who have previously expressed suicidal ideation or made suicide attempts, or those with mood disorders or substance abuse disorders, who are higher risk than the general population.

Mental health treatment is typically organized into biological therapies, including both pharmacotherapy (e.g., antidepressants), and electroconvulsive therapy (ECT), and psychosocial approaches, such as psychotherapy (e.g., cognitive-behavioral therapy), supportive counseling or treatment for substance abuse.

Because suicide attempts are known to be a strong predictor of future attempts (and completions), specific invention efforts have been directed to this high-risk population. Typically this involves tracking individuals after emergency room visits for suicide attempts, providing close mental health follow up, therapy, or case management.

Restriction of access to lethal means covers a variety of population-wide measures that limit the availability of commonly used methods of suicide. These include restricting access to highly lethal means (firearms through background checks, waiting periods, licensing laws, or bans, jumping by installing barriers on bridges), common means (limiting package sizes or configurations of pharmaceuticals used in overdose, most commonly acetaminophen), and other community or social interventions (such as changing the source and composition of domestic gas to have a lower carbon monoxide content, and requiring the installation of catalytic converters on all newly manufactured vehicles to reduce the level of carbon monoxide in the exhaust gas). An important issue in means restriction is whether reducing the availability of one mechanism will reduce the suicide rate overall, or merely shift suicides towards other available methods.

Media reporting guidelines are designed to address the problem of imitation or contagion: widely publicized suicides, especially of celebrities, are thought to temporarily increase the suicide rate, especially of suicides that mimic the reported mechanism. More information about the media and imitative suicides can be found in a recent review by Pirkis.[8].

Suicide prevention programs, especially those designed for very large organizations such as military forces, or for entire nations, are typically multifaceted programs comprising a variety of different interventions just mentioned; most often the multifaceted programs combine population-based programs that use education and screening with more targeted interventions for those with identified risk factors.

Other factors not explicitly listed above, such as substance abuse, and homelessness, are also relevant because they affect impulsivity or hopelessness, and are also obvious targets of both mental health and broader social interventions.

Because completed suicide is a very rare event in small samples, various approaches have been taken in assessing the efficacy of intervention programs. First, intermediate or proxy outcome measures can be used. Relevant outcomes would be decreases in depression rating scores, or decreased reports of suicidal ideation. However, the use of these measure greatly inflates the number of implicated studies for review – the examples mentioned would involve nearly all the published literature on the treatment of mood disorders – or involve subjective assessments of the strength of the suicidal ideation and whether the ideation was the precursor of an intended act or merely a means of communication to others or of obtaining hospital admission. Because of these concerns, the outcomes used in this report are suicide attempts, and completed suicides.

In this report we review the state of the evidence for suicide prevention, with a special focus on the military and veteran populations. The interventions are organized into the taxonomy presented above. The three key questions were:

1. What are the new or improved suicide prevention strategies (e.g. hotlines, outreach programs, peer counseling, treatment coordination programs, and new counseling approaches) that show promise for Veterans?

2. What solid evidence base supports the most promising strategies?

3. What evidence is still needed to establish various strategies as the most promising (framed as research questions to guide and focus continued research to expand knowledge regarding the effectiveness of suicide prevention approaches)?

METHODS

TOPIC DEVELOPMENT

This project was nominated by the Office of Research and Development for the Evidence Synthesis Project. Key questions were discussed and finalized during a conference call that included the Steering Committee of the Evidence Synthesis Project and the VA Greater Los Angeles project site director. The final key questions are:

1. What are the new or improved suicide prevention strategies (e.g. hotlines, outreach programs, peer counseling, treatment coordination programs, and new counseling approaches) that show promise for Veterans?

2. What solid evidence base supports the most promising strategies?

3. What evidence is still needed to establish various strategies as the most promising (framed as research questions to guide and focus continued research to expand knowledge regarding the effectiveness of suicide prevention approaches)?

SEARCH STRATEGY

Mann et al. completed a systematic review of the literature on suicide prevention from 1966 through June 2005.[1] As we scored this article well on those aspects of the Oxman-Guyatt Overview Quality Assessment Questionnaire[9] and the AMSTAR Systematic Review Checklist[10] that dealt with the rigor of the search and selection process, we judged the articles identified by this review as a suitable starting place for our own review. They searched MEDLINE, the Cochrane Library, and PsychINFO databases. We updated this using the same search strategy, starting from July 2005 through May 2008.

The search strategy is listed below:

DATABASES SEARCHED & TIME PERIOD COVERED:
PubMed
June 2005 – May 2008

LIMITERS: ENGLISH

SEARCH STRATEGY:
Suicide/prevention and control
OR
suicide, attempted/prevention and control
OR
suicide AND (prevent*[tiab] OR depression OR health education
OR health promotion OR public opinion OR mass screening OR
family physicians OR medical education OR primary health care
OR antidepressive agents OR psychotherapy OR schools OR
adolescents OR methods OR firearms OR overdose OR poisoning
OR gas poisoning OR mass media)
NOT
case report* OR editorial* OR letter

TOTAL RESULTS – 3,212[+]

[+]references to "suicide cells" & "suicide genes" were manually removed and are not included in
this number

In addition to our PubMed search, we performed reference mining of retrieved articles,
references of prior reviews, and solicited articles from experts.

STUDY SELECTION

In consultation with the ESP Advisory Committee and VA policymakers in mental health, we
developed the following criteria to guide study selection. Our focus was on veterans and active
military duty persons, consequently studies of children and adolescents were excluded. All
studies of veterans and military personnel (from any country) were included. In addition to this,
we included studies of the non-veteran population from the US and countries sufficiently similar
to the US in terms of culture (Canada, United Kingdom, Ireland, Australia, New Zealand). Only
studies that reported outcomes as suicides or suicide attempts were included; studies reporting
only other proxy outcomes were excluded. Studies of strictly mental health interventions
(psychotherapy, pharmacotherapy) have been reviewed by others and were therefore excluded
unless they included military or veterans.

DATA ABSTRACTION

Data were abstracted by a psychiatrist with prior experience in systematic reviews. The following data were abstracted from included trials: population, mean and median age, setting, country, interventions, outcomes, and study design. Data abstraction forms are provided in Appendix A.

QUALITY ASSESSMENT OF INDIVIDUAL ARTICLES

To assess the quality of the RCT and CCTs we used was a modification of the Delphi List.[11] We abstracted data on whether or not the study was described as randomized; treatment allocation; was the method of randomization performed and was the treatment allocation concealed; were the groups similar at baseline regarding the most important prognostic indicators; were the eligibility criteria specified; was the outcome assessor blinded; was the care provider blinded; was the patient blinded; were point estimates and measures of variability presented for the primary outcome measures; were all randomized participants analyzed in the group to which they were allocated; were co-interventions avoided or similar; was compliance in all groups acceptable; was the timing of the outcome assessment in all groups similar.

RATING THE BODY OF EVIDENCE

We assessed the overall quality of evidence for outcomes using a method developed by the Grade Working Group, which classified the grade of evidence across outcomes according to the following criteria:[12]
- **High** = Further research is very unlikely to change our confidence on the estimate of effect.
- **Moderate** = Further research is likely to have an important impact on our confidence in the estimate of effect and may change the estimate.
- **Low** = Further research is very likely to have an important impact on our confidence in the estimate of effect and is likely to change the estimate.
- **Very Low** = Any estimate of effect is very uncertain.

GRADE also suggests using the following scheme for assigning the "grade" or strength of evidence:

Criteria for assigning grade of evidence

Type of evidence
Randomized trial = high
Observational study = low
Any other evidence = very low

Decrease grade if:
- Serious (-1) or very serious (-2) limitation to study quality
- Important inconsistency (-1)
- Some (-1) or major (-2) uncertainty about directness
- Imprecise or sparse data (-1)
- High probability of reporting bias (-1)

Increase grade if:
- Strong evidence of association-significant relative risk of > 2 (< 0.5) based on consistent evidence from two or more observational studies, with no plausible confounders (+1)
- Very strong evidence of association-significant relative risk of > 5 (< 0.2) based on direct evidence with no major threats to validity (+2)
- Evidence of a dose response gradient (+1)
- All plausible confounders would have reduced the effect (+1)

For this report, we used both this explicit scoring scheme and the global implicit judgment about "confidence" in the result. Where the two disagreed, we went with the lower of the two classifications.

DATA SYNTHESIS

The studies included in this review were too heterogeneous to statistically pool, and we therefore summarized these narratively, in the following categories multifaceted interventions for military personnel; other multifaceted programs (national suicide prevention programs); interventions for veterans; psychosocial interventions post-suicide attempt; postal or telephone follow up post-suicide attempt; hospital admission for attempted suicide; and restriction of access to lethal means.

PEER REVIEW

This report was reviewed by 6 experts selected by the VA ESP Advisory Committee for their expertise in this area and their knowledge of VA. Peer review comments received, and the changes we made to the report as a result, are presented in Appendix D.

RESULTS

LITERATURE FLOW – UPDATE

In total, we examined 3,406 titles. The electronic literature search identified 3,212 articles. An additional 196 articles were identified through reference mining. A content expert identified 5 more articles.

Of the titles identified through our electronic literature search, 3,140 were rejected at title review as clearly irrelevant to the project. This left 273 from all sources. Seven articles were rejected as not relevant. Five titles could not be located after contacting many sources. (Figure 2)

We reviewed a total of 261 articles. Initial screening of the articles resulted in three articles that included veterans and seven articles that included military personnel. We excluded 135 article for the following reasons: five because they did not include an intervention, two foreign language articles, three articles contained duplicate data, 41 review or meta-analyses, 82 articles with no outcome of interest or no usable data, one study of adolescents only, and one editorial. This left 126 articles included for further review.

Following guidance from the ESP Advisory Committee in our further inclusion criteria we excluded an additional 49 studies. Studies were excluded for studies conducted in countries other than US, Canada, United Kingdom, Ireland, Australia, or New Zealand and not containing military personnel or veterans; only reporting suicidal ideations, or being a strictly psychotherapy or pharmacotherapy study. Of studies that met our inclusion criteria we found 20 RCT or CCT studies, 28 observational studies, 6 cohort studies, and 23 interrupted time series studies.

Excluded articles and reasons for exclusion are listed in Appendix B.

The results have been grouped together by the kind of intervention, and within that, by study design. We first report on studies of military or veterans that use multifaceted (multi-component) interventions. This includes all the studies (of any type) that directly studied military personnel. For comparison, we then present other multifaceted interventions, both of which are national suicide prevention programs. We then report on several other interventions identified that included veterans.

13

Figure 2. Literature Flow

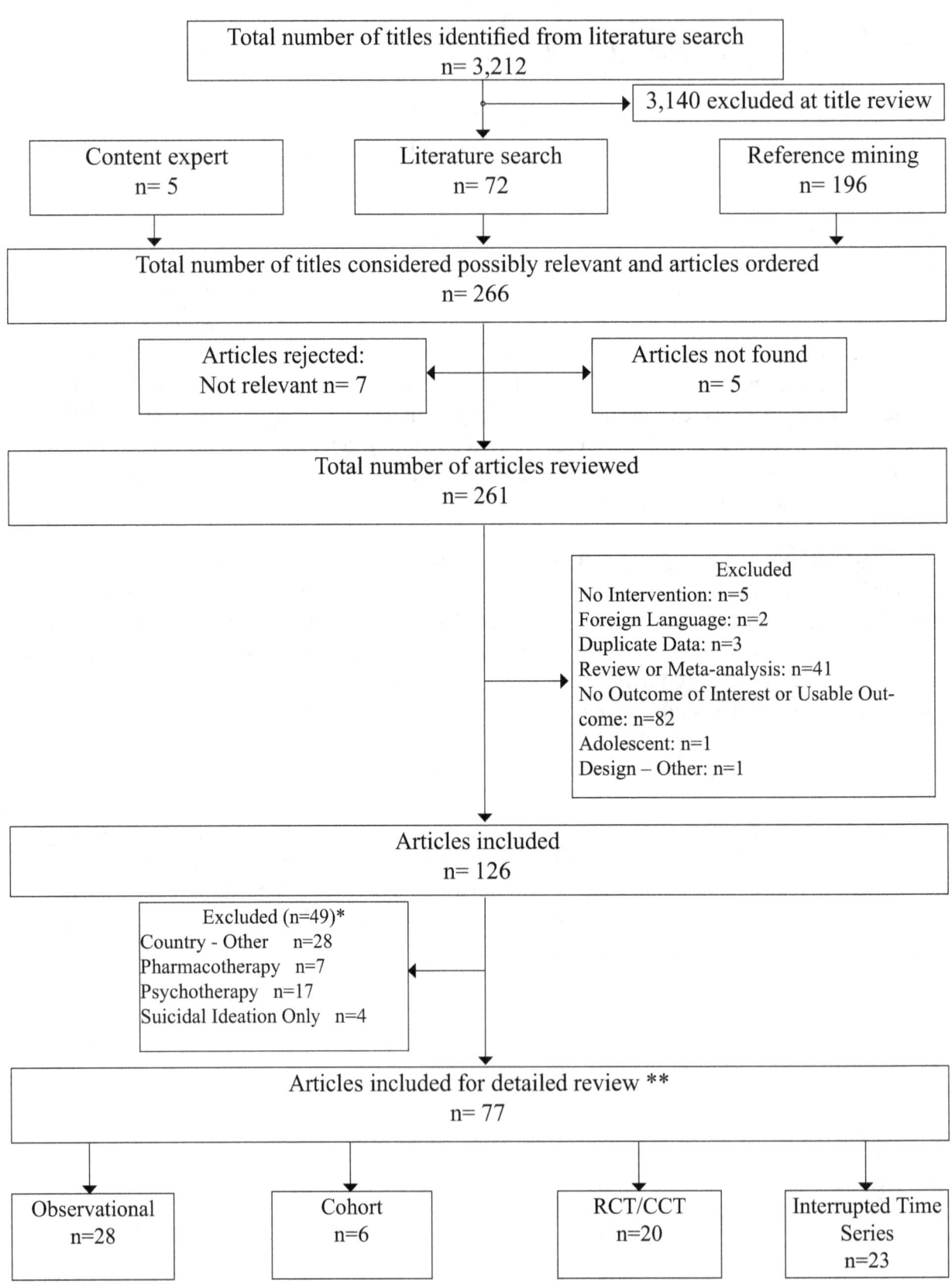

Total number of titles identified from literature search
n= 3,212

→ 3,140 excluded at title review

Content expert
n= 5

Literature search
n= 72

Reference mining
n= 196

Total number of titles considered possibly relevant and articles ordered
n= 266

Articles rejected:
Not relevant n= 7

Articles not found
n= 5

Total number of articles reviewed
n= 261

Excluded
No Intervention: n=5
Foreign Language: n=2
Duplicate Data: n=3
Review or Meta-analysis: n=41
No Outcome of Interest or Usable Outcome: n=82
Adolescent: n=1
Design – Other: n=1

Articles included
n= 126

Excluded (n=49)*
Country - Other   n=28
Pharmacotherapy   n=7
Psychotherapy   n=17
Suicidal Ideation Only   n=4

Articles included for detailed review **
n= 77

Observational
n=28

Cohort
n=6

RCT/CCT
n=20

Interrupted Time
Series
n=23

*Studies excluded for multiple reasons

KEY QUESTION #1: What are the new or improved suicide prevention strategies (e.g. hotlines, outreach programs, peer counseling, treatment coordination programs, and new counseling approaches) that show promise for Veterans?

KEY QUESTION #2: What solid evidence base supports the most promising strategies?

OVERVIEW

This results section is organized by the target and the method of the intervention, first with studies of multifaceted interventions. We found studies of multifaceted interventions only for military personnel or the general population. We did not find any studies of multifaceted interventions for veterans. Following the review of multifaceted interventions is a review of the studies that did include veterans. The report then discusses evidence from other populations using interventions post-suicide attempt, suicide prevention centers, hospital admission for attempted suicide, collaborative care for depression, and an intervention for the identified patient's support network. Then observational studies for restricting access to lethal means (firearms, acetaminophen, other toxic agents, and bridge barriers), and restrictions of media reporting of suicides are presented.

Multifaceted interventions for military personnel

Seven studies involving military personnel were identified. All were prospective cohort studies in which the intervention was implemented for the entire population. The characteristics, interventions, and outcomes of the military studies are shown in Evidence Table 1 in Appendix C.

James and Kowalski[13] described a suicide prevention program for the US Army 25th Infantry Division (Light) that was started in 1992 and fully implemented by early 1994. Psychological autopsy data from 1985 to 1993 identified various risk factors in this population including demographics (all male), mental status (depression), substance abuse, and relationship problems (all the suicides involved marital or relationship discord or alleged infidelity). The intervention reported was multifactorial and multidisciplinary. The disciplines involved included the chaplain (to provide individual counseling and division-wide education), the psychologist (to coordinate training, and assist in identifying high-risk soldiers), the social worker (to provide a liaison for the soldier, their family, and the soldier's commander). Specific components of the intervention as reported included: lectures by chaplains, lectures at training programs (for division commanders and enlisted soldiers), pocket-sized cards with warning signs and contact information for emergency services, "crisis-intervention command consultations" (special meetings with soldier, their commanders, and division mental health officer), a "high-risk book" (once identified as high risk, the soldier's commander provide bi-monthly written assessments on the soldier's progress), outpatient follow up care with mental health services, and mental health services for the soldier and their family, along with a substance abuse prevention program. The size of the study population was not reported. The program was not formally evaluated, but in a postscript the authors noted, "the suicide rate has decreased to three in the past 2 years." Unfortunately, the baseline comparison rate was not clearly reported, so we cannot reach any conclusions about effectiveness.

McDaniel et al.[14] reported on a suicide prevention program at a US Navy Training Command that was implemented after a cluster of suicides in 1986. The target of the intervention was the petty officers and chief petty officers who were the instructors at the command. They were educated to recognize risk factors likely to be common in the students of the training command (recent interpersonal losses, substance abuse, social isolation, and personality disorders and psychiatric illnesses), and about the goals of fostering group cohesiveness and ensuring treatment compliance for those referred for treatment. The size of the study population was not reported. The main outcome assessed was suicide attempts at the training command in comparison with that reported at a similarly sized operational command nearby. They reported a statistically significant negative correlation between the number of instructors trained and the number of suicide attempts. They concluded that the program reduced the number of suicide attempts at the training command. However, there were a number of complicating factors, including seasonal factors stemming for start dates for cohorts of students at the training command and limited of hours of operation when potentially suicidal students were referred to the operational command for evaluation (thus inflating the number of suicide attempts reported at the latter facility).

Knox et al.[15] described a multifactorial suicide prevention program implemented in the US Air Force, comprising over 5,000,000 active duty personnel. The intervention was designed to reduce stigma and risk factors, and strengthen protective factors in a population-based approach. The program had 11 components. There was training for squadron commanders, addition of suicide prevention into required training, use of guidelines for mental health referral, addition of staff to support community-based preventive services at mental health centers, and required training for non-professionals in suicide risks and referral procedures. The program also assessed for suicide risk those under investigation for legal problems, established teams to respond to traumatic events including suicides, integrated the delivery system for human services prevention activities, established patient privilege in psychotherapy, conducted a behavior health survey, and established a suicide event surveillance system for tracking risk factors. To evaluate the program, the USAF population from 1990-6 was the control cohort, and the 1997-2002 population was the treatment cohort. No differences in demographic characteristics or in rates for mental health disability were found between the two groups. There was a statistically significant trend for decline in suicide rate over time, with a 33% reduction of risk for completed suicide compared to the baseline rate. The average rate in the pre-intervention period was 13.5 per 100,000, and 9.2 in the post-intervention period.

Jones et al.[16] described a US Navy and Marine Corps initiative to reducing suicide using "best practice strategies." They identified existing resources relevant to suicide prevention, which included awareness (education about suicide prevention for all personnel and in leadership schools), life skills training (for substance abuse, stress and anger management, conflict resolution), post-suicide attempt interventions (family support, critical event stress debriefing), and data collection (suicide incident reports with explicit monitoring and tracking of data). A training video on suicide prevention was developed for all personnel; it highlighted positive role models and early identification of those at risk by co-workers, and was included as part of the required annual General Military Training (GMT) starting in the summer of 2000. The size of the study population was not reported. The authors reported that, "the introduction of annual suicide prevention GMT requirement coincided with a drop in Navy suicide rate for FY-01 to 9.2/100K. This is the lowest rate in 10 years." The Marine Corps rate for the same year was 15.6/100,000, but no baseline rate or comparison was provided.

Kennedy et al.[17] described an overseas gambling treatment program for the US Navy. Pathological gambling was recognized to have significant psychiatric comorbidity, including substance abuse, mood disorders, and suicidality. The program focused on overseas gambling because of the relative lack of restriction on slot machines in military clubs overseas, and the lack of overseas treatment options for pathological gambling. The services were provided at a naval base in Okinawa, Japan within the context of a substance abuse rehabilitation program, and included psychological evaluation, individual and group counseling, patient and family education, Gambler's Anonymous, and access to a gambling crisis counseling around the clock. The program was evaluated for a year (roughly, the calendar year 2004) during which 35 individuals were referred. Twenty percent of those reported suicidal ideation, and 3 had made gambling-related suicide attempts before referral. During the treatment period, there were no attempted suicides and no suicidal ideation recurred.

Two suicide military-based suicide prevention programs outside the US have been reported. Rozanov et al.[18] described a program implemented in a military unit of size 10,000 in the Ukrainian Army. The program set up training seminars about suicide, risk factors, and prevention for commanders, officers, and basic soldiers. Training booklets were also distributed. The suicide rates in the years 1988-1999 (pre-implementation) were compared to the rates in 2000 and 2001. The total suicide rate over all military personnel in the pre-implementation period was 32.6 per 100,000. The rate for 2000 was 0 and 16.7 for 2001.

Gordana and Milivoje[19] reported on a suicide prevention program in the Army of Serbia and Montenegro, influenced by the USAF program of Knox,[15] above. The program components included selection (to remove recruits with serious mental problems), education about suicide risk factors, and motivation for military duty. Training was provided to soldiers about maladjustment and substance abuse. Unit and central command physicians, psychologists, and officers were also involved. The program was fully implemented in December 2003. The size of the study population was not reported. The annual suicide rate for the Yugoslav Army for the years 1999 to 2003 was 13 per 100,000, declining in the post-implementation period to 5 per 100,000 in 2004.

In summary, seven studies of suicide prevention for military personnel were identified. All used a conceptual model of risk factor identification, based on review of suicides in the population under study, augmented with factors previously identified by others, followed by educational and organizational changes to reduce those factors or increase education and awareness about them. All were multifaceted programs, and all reported declines in suicides or suicide attempts.

However, the reporting of sufficient data to make proper comparison was incomplete, and the quality of the analysis that was reported was generally poor. The largest studies were deployed for the US Navy and Marine Corps and for the US Air Force. The clearly methodologically strongest study was that of Knox et al.[15] for the US Air Force, which also appears to have influenced other studies. However, much more data are needed in order to better understand what are the most effective components to include in a multicomponent intervention, and how each component can be both internally optimized and made most synergistic with the other components.

Other multifaceted programs (national suicide prevention programs)

Two studies reporting results of multicomponent national suicide prevention programs were identified, one for Australia, and one for England. Both were prospective, cohort designs.

Robinson et al.[20] published a commentary on Australia's National Suicide Prevention Strategy. They divided the interventions in the NSPS into universal (targeting populations), selective (groups with risk factors), and indicated (for groups that have already displayed some suicidal thoughts or behaviors). Most of the interventions were universal interventions aimed at young people or minorities. They noted that neither those with mental illness nor those with previous suicide attempts had been the targets of any of the national initiatives. During the interval of the program's existence, 1999 to 2004, the suicide rate dropped from 22 to 17 for men, and 5 to 4 for women, both measured per 100,000. As they note, this decline "cannot necessarily be attributed to the NSPS."

In 2002, England started a national suicide prevention program, the status of which has been documented in a series of yearly updates, the latest of which covers through year 2006.[21] Their multifaceted program includes mental health (focus on post-hospital discharge and non-compliance with treatment), study of self-harm as a risk for suicide, mental health promotion projects for young men and for those in the prison system. Their program also includes efforts to reduce access to lethal means (removing points for hanging on psychiatric wards, and a phased withdrawal of co-proxamol, a painkiller lethal in overdose), and establishment of systems to conduct suicide audits through Primary Care Trusts. The program set a target of a 20% reduction in suicides during the implementation period. Using age-standardized rates, the rate for 2003-5 was compared the baseline rate for 1995-7. The post-intervention rate was 8.5 deaths per 100,000, which represented at 7.4% decrease from the baseline rate.

In summary, two national suicide prevention programs reported declines in suicide rates coincident with the introduction of those programs. Both published reports provided scant details on methodology.

Interventions for veterans

Three reports involving US veterans were identified. This is a heterogeneous set. One was an RCT using psychotherapy for female veterans with borderline personality disorder. One study looked at the association between treatment in a residential program for substance abuse and suicide attempts. One study examined the association between treatment with antidepressant medication and the development of suicidal ideation. (Evidence tables for RCT/CCTs in this section and subsequent sections are shown in Evidence Table 2, which includes the quality assessment ratings; all Military/Veteran Studies are shown in Evidence Table 1)

Koons et al.[22] reported a pilot RCT of dialectical behavior therapy for female veterans with borderline personality disorder. Patients with the appropriate diagnosis were recruited through clinics at the Durham VA and other VA clinics in North Carolina. The treatment group received dialectical behavior therapy, a kind of psychotherapy explicitly designed to treat patients with chronic suicidality or self-injurious behaviors. It includes both individual and group therapy, and separate consultation sessions for the therapists, all conducted weekly. The treatment lasted 6 months. The control group received weekly individual therapy. The assessed outcome was intentional self-harm (including suicide attempts) in the preceding 3 months. In the treatment group this decreased from 50% to 10% (at 6 months), and in the control group decreased from 30% to 20%. This decrease was not statistically significant, possibly due to the small sample size (10 patients completed in each group).

Ilgen[23] studied US veterans entering substance abuse treatment programs (either residential or outpatient), and compared the suicide attempt rate in the previous 12 months at program entry, during treatment, and in the 12 month follow-up interval. The median treatment duration was 12 months. A total of 3733 patients were followed. In predicting suicide attempts during treatment, residential treatment was associated with a lower rate than outpatient treatment, even when baseline suicidality was controlled for. In predicting suicide attempts after treatment, none of treatment setting (residential vs. outpatient), availability of psychiatric services, and use of psychiatric services was statistically significant, although longer treatment episode was.

Gibbons et al.[24] examined the hypothesized association between treatment with antidepressants and the development of suicidal ideation and behavior; earlier studies had led to the FDA's black box warning for children, adolescents, and young adults for these medications. The authors studied administrative and pharmacy data from the Veteran Health Administration with data on over 226000 patients to identify those patients with new depressive disorders (no history in the prior two years). The outcome variable was suicide attempts treated at VA facilities. Cause of death information was not available for completed suicides. When compared to those depressed patients not receiving an antidepressant, there were reductions in the suicide rate for each class (SSRI monotherapy, non-SSRI monotherapy, and tricyclic monotherapy) studies. When suicide attempt rates were compared within in each class of treatment, the relative risk (in treatment vs. before treatment) was reduced with treatment.

In summary, three studies involving US veterans. One RCT found a trend not reaching statistical significant for the use of dialectical behavior therapy for female veterans with borderline personality disorder. One reported mixed results looking at associations between residential treatment of substance abuse and suicide attempts. One reported reduction in suicide rates associated with treatment with antidepressants. Because of the study designs, it was not possible to infer causality from the reported associations, and the heterogeneity of these studies limits any generalization.

Psychosocial interventions post-suicide attempt

Twelve studies were found that described case management or therapeutic interventions initiated after presentations for suicide attempts. These studies are presented here by country, and then chronologically.

Psychosocial interventions post-suicide attempt, USA

Welu[25] described a program implemented for those making a suicide attempt seen in the emergency room of a hospital in Pittsburgh, Pennsylvania. Patients in the treatment group were seen in a special outreach program staffed by registered nurses, social workers, and community workers. Patients were contacted as soon as possible after release from the hospital to set up home visits. Subsequently mental health treatment designed to meet the needs of that particular patient were made available. Patients were in contact with staff at least biweekly to provide treatment, or to monitor the treatment when it was provided by other services. Patients assigned to the control group were treated in the usual manner in the ER or hospital, and released with written appointments; no attempts were made to provide outreach to those who failed to follow up. Patients were randomized to the treatment or control group. Both groups were contacted for an interview 4 months after the suicide attempt for assessment. The outcome was the number of suicide reattempts in the 4 month follow up period. The treatment group had 4.8% reattempt rate, while the control group had a 15.8% reattempt rate, a statistically significant difference.

Psychosocial interventions post-suicide attempt, Canada

Termansen and Bywater[26] described a project implemented at Vancouver General Hospital for all patients presenting to that emergency room for a suicide attempt during a three month period in 1972. Patients were allocated to one of four treatment groups on a rotating (nonrandom) basis. The first group was assessed in the ER and followed for three months for the same (lay) mental health worker. The second group was assessed in the ER by a mental health worker, but followed by a crisis center volunteer for three months and then assessed by that volunteer and a mental health worker. The third group received the ER assessment by the mental health worked but with no follow up other than assessment at three months. The fourth group was identified on the basis of ER records, received no other intervention, and was assessed at three months by a mental health worker. The follow up provided to the first two groups was either in-person or by phone on a schedule of decreasing frequency from daily for the first week down to every other week for weeks 9 through 12. They reported the number of suicide attempts in each group: Group 1 had 1/45 (2.2%), Group 2 had 2/33 (6.1%), Group 3 had 7/32 (22%), and Group 4 had 2/18 (11.1%). The lower rate for Group 1 was statistically significant.

Allard et al.[27] reported on a follow-up program used in several Montreal hospitals after a suicide attempt. The treatment group received an intensive intervention program consisting of an explicit treatment plan, a schedule of visits for a year, at least one home visit from a social worker, appointment reminders by phone or in writing or home visits for missed appointments, and referral for normal psychiatric treatment at the end of the one-year program. Specific mental health treatment was left to the therapist and could include biologic or psychotherapeutic treatment. The control group received normal care at the hospital. Patients were randomized to the treatment or control group. The outcome assessed was the recurrence of suicide attempts in the two years following the index attempt. They found a recurrence rate of 35% in the treatment group, and 30% in the control group, a statistically insignificant difference. There were three suicide completions in the treatment group and one in the control group.

Psychosocial interventions post-suicide attempt, UK

Chowdhury et al.[28] described an experimental program at the Regional Poisoning Treatment Centre in Edinburgh, Scotland, for those making repeated suicide attempts, defined as those with a history of one or more prior admissions to that facility within the previous three years. The treatment was a new service staffed by mental health clinicians that offered follow up care in local clinics (either scheduled, or in a walk-in basis), with home visits for all those patients who did not keep scheduled appointments. Arrangements were also made so that patients calling a local suicide hotline would be called by staff, scheduled for an appointment, or seen at home by the service staff. Eligible patients were alternately (not randomly) assigned to either the treatment group or the control group, the latter group receiving the usual treatment of being scheduled with a mental health clinician, but with no attempts to pursue those who failed to keep the appointment. An exception was made for those patients judged to be at high risk of suicide; these patients were automatically assigned to the treatment service, but excluded from the treatment group for comparison in the analysis. The reported outcome was the number of suicide attempts in a six-month follow up period. They found that 24% of the treatment group patients and 23% of the control group patients had one or more suicide attempts, a statistically insignificant difference by the chi-squared test. There were no completed suicides in either group.

Gardner et al.[29] reported on a suicide-attempt evaluation program implemented at a hospital in Cambridge, England. All patients admitted for a self-poisoning were randomly assigned for assessment to either a medical team (including a social worker) or a psychiatrist. The medical team members received some (unspecified) instruction in psychiatric evaluation. The purpose of the assessment was to determine whether further inpatient or outpatient psychiatric care was needed. Patients were followed for one year after their attempt. Patient who re-presented at the hospital with subsequent attempts were reentered into the study and re-randomized to an intervention; these patients were thus counted more than once. The outcomes assessed were reattempts or completions. Survival curves for the proportion of admissions without relapse (reattempt) were constructed, and showed a slight but not statistically significant trend for less relapse for those patients assigned to the medical team. A similar result was found when using only first-admission data for each patient. There were no suicides in the medical team group and one suicide in the psychiatrist group.

Gibbons et al.[30] reported on a post-suicide social work intervention program at Southampton General Hospital, England. The treatment was a "task-centered casework" approach, in which specific problems in social roles, transitions, or resources were identified, and set out as tasks that the social worker helped the client complete. These services were provided in the patients' homes. Patient who presented to the hospital Accident and Emergency Department (ER) with deliberate self-poisonings were randomly assigned to either the treatment or the control group of routine treatment (referral back to General Practitioner or to psychiatry). The outcome assessed was the number of recurrences of self-poisoning in the 12 months after the index attempt. The treatment group had 13.5% recurrence rate, while the control group had a 14.5% recurrence rate, a statistically insignificant difference.

Hawton et al.[31] reported on a domiciliary (home-based) treatment program for patients admitted to the General Hospital in Oxford, England for deliberate self-poisoning. A special service for such patients was developed using nursing and social work staff, using a problem-oriented crisis intervention approach. In this study the treatment group received these services at home as often as the therapists felt necessary. The control group received the same services provided weekly in clinic. Treatment in both groups lasted up to 3 months. Patients were randomly assigned to either the treatment or control group. The outcome measure was the rate of repetition of suicide attempt. They found the domiciliary group had a repetition rate of 10%, and the out-patient group a rate of 15% in the year following the index overdose. This difference was not statistically significant.

Hawton et al.[32] described a program comparing out-patient counseling with referral to General Practitioner care for patients admitted to the General Hospital in Oxford, England for deliberate self-poisoning. The treatment group was given out-patient counseling using a problem-oriented approach by the clinician who conducted the initial assessment. The meaning of the attempt was explored, and alternative coping mechanisms were identified. In the control group patients were referred back to their GPs with recommendations for further care, such as marital therapy. Patients were randomized to the treatment or control group. The outcome assessed was the rate of repeated suicide attempt at one year post-attempt. The treatment group had a 15.4% repeat rate, while the control group had a 7.3% repeat rate; this difference was not statistically significant. There was one completed suicide in the out-patient counseling group; "she had attended OP counseling sessions, but before the end of treatment moved to another area where she was referred to psychiatric care, and where her death occurred."

Guthrie et al.[33] reported on a brief psychological intervention after deliberate self-poisoning implemented at a hospital in Manchester, England. The treatment consisted of four sessions of psychodynamic interpersonal therapy, starting within a week of presentation at the hospital's emergency department. The therapy was given by a nurse in the patient's home. The control group was given routine care, which involved assessment in the ER and referral to psychiatry, addiction services, or their general practitioner. Patients were randomized to the treatment or control group. The outcome assessed was further episodes of self-harm within a six-month period. The treatment group had a 9% repeat rate, while the control group had a 28% repeat rate, a statistically significant decrease. There were no completed suicides in either group.

Bennewith et al.[34] conducted a cluster randomized controlled trial of a general practice-based intervention in a region of England. For practices include in the treatment group, new episodes of self-harm in patients of those practices were identified. If the episode was the first for that patient during the trial period, the patient's general practitioner was sent a letter informing them of the incident, along with another letter to forward to the patient inviting the patient to schedule an appointment, and a copy of treatment guidelines for the management of self harm to be placed in the patient's chart and used during their appointment. The control group received normal referral services. GP practices were randomized to the treatment or control group. The outcome assessed was the recurrence of an episode of deliberate self-harm in the 12 months after the index episode. The treatment group had a recurrence rate of 21.9%, while the control group had a recurrence rate of 19.5%; this difference was not statistically significant. Time to the repeat episode and the number of repeat episodes were also not statistically significantly different.

Clarke et al.[35] reported on an intervention for deliberate self-harm, implemented at two Accident & Emergency (ER) departments on the London/Essex border in England. The intervention group received case management services from a nurse practitioner who conducted an initial assessment, constructed a care plan, and was available on a 'open access' basis by mobile phone; the NP coordinated access to care but did not provide the services themselves. The intervention group also received the routine care provided to the control group, which comprised triage services and medical and psychiatric treatment as needed. Patients were randomized to the treatment or control group. The outcome assessed was the readmission rate for recurrent self-harm. In the 12 months following the index episode, the treatment group had a 9% readmission rate, while the control group had a 10% readmission rate; this difference was not statistically significant. A statistically significant greater number of patients requiring multiple readmissions were in the treatment group.

Psychosocial interventions post-suicide attempt, Australia

Aoun[36] described a non-randomized intervention in a region of Western Australia. All patients presenting at one particular hospital or to community clinics after a suicide attempt or who were judged to be at risk of self-harm were offered the intervention. The intervention consisted of a suicide intervention counselor who provided crisis management and coordination of follow-up out to 6 weeks from first contact. Patients could be referred to GPs, other health professionals and agencies. The hospital also enhanced assessment and treatment while in the hospital, and the suicide intervention counselor provided education about risk assessment and treatment resources to health professionals and the community. A 2 year pre-intervention retrospective chart review was conducted to establish the baseline outcomes. Information on the program was collected for 22 months starting in November 1995. The outcome assessed with the number of suicide attempts leading to readmission. Those in the treatment group had a reattempt rate of 3.6%, while those in the standard treatment group had a reattempt rate of 12.6%; this was statistically significant. The pre-intervention rate in the preceding 22 months was 11.1%; this was statistically significant when compared to the treatment group rate. The author did note that during the treatment period the total number of hospital admissions increased; this appears to have been in part driven by a policy to hospitalize for assessment and treatment.

In summary, 12 studies, nearly all randomized or controlled clinical trials, reporting psychosocial interventions post-suicide attempt were identified. Interventions varied, but mostly consisted of additional resources, such as case management to monitor patients, and facilitate access to mental health services. Most studies did not report any statistically significant differences between treatment and control, and in many the proportion of repeat attempts were within a few percent of other. In other studies the average difference was 5%-8% indicating a signal of potential efficacy that possibly could be detected with a larger sample size. The four studies reporting statistically significant results did not differ in any marked way from the nonsignificant studies in terms of patients studied, interventions, or study quality. However, a wide range in suicide attempt rates across studies was noted. The efficacy of these programs does not appear to be robust, and it remains what program characteristics led to the positive results in those four studies, and indeed unclear whether psychosocial interventions aimed at suicide attempters reduce repeated attempts.

Postal or telephone follow up post-suicide attempt

Four studies reporting on telephone or postal follow up after suicide attempts were identified. They are presented by country and then by date.

Postal or telephone follow up post-suicide attempt, USA

Motto and Bostrom[37] described a program in San Francisco for patients admitted to a psychiatric hospital for depression or "suicidal state." All patients were offered post-discharge therapy. All patients who declined such treatment or discontinued within 30 days were then randomized to either the contact group or the no-contact group. Patients in the contact group received short, personalized letters from the research staff who had conducted their initial interviews expressing concern about the patient, and inviting the patient to respond if they desired. No specific recommendations or treatments were made in the letters. Letters were sent monthly for four months, every two months for eight months, and every three months for four years for a total of 24 contacts over 5 years. Patients in the no-contact group and those who had complied with the initial post-discharge therapy received no letters. The outcome assessed was completed suicides. In five years after the index contact, the treatment (contact) group had a suicide rate of 3.9% compared to the control (no-contact) group at 4.6%. These rates at 15 years were 6.4% for treatment and 5.7% for control. A survival analysis showed statistically significant differences for the first two years, but not later. They concluded that the results were consistent with their study hypothesis: that the period of maximum contact, especially the first year, would have the greater divergence in suicide rate.

Postal or telephone follow up post-suicide attempt, UK

Morgan et al.[38] reported an intervention to provide patients seen in the Accident and Emergency (ER) department for first episodes of deliberate self-harm with easy access by phone to on-call trainee psychiatrists. This study was conducted in the United Bristol Healthcare Trust catchment area in England. Specifically, those in the treatment group were provided a 'green card' which stated that a doctor was available at all times by telephone, and also encouraged patients to seek care by phone or in person at the ER. Those assigned to the treatment group received another copy of the card by mail at their home address three weeks after the index episode. Their GPs were also sent a copy of the card and asked to discuss it with the patients as appropriate. The control group received routine care. Patients were randomized to the treatment or control group.

The outcome assessed was the repetition of deliberate self-harm. There were 7 repeats in the treatment group, and 15 repeats in the control group. No completed suicides occurred in either group. Measures of statistical significance were not reported.

Evans et al.[39] repeated the study of Morgan et al.[38] with the same intervention, modified to allow patients with previous episodes of self-harm, and providing them only phone contact without offers of in-person assessment or hospital admission. Patients were again randomized to the treatment or control group. The rate of repetition of deliberate self-harm in the treatment group was 16.8% compared to 14.4% in the control group. This difference was not statistically significant. There were two completed suicides in the treatment group and one suicide in the control group. They noted that "neither of the suicides from the green card group had made use of the green card at any time to seek help."

Postal or telephone follow up post-suicide attempt, Australia

Carter et al.[40] implemented a postcard-based intervention, based on the Motto and Bostrom[37] study, for those patients with deliberate self-poisoning presenting at regional toxicology unit in New South Wales, Australia. The intervention consisted of a postcard sent to the patient in a sealed envelope at 1, 2, 3,4, 6, 8, 10, and 12 months post-discharge. The card wished the patient well and invited a response if they were interested. The control treatment was not described. Patients were randomized to the treatment or control group. The outcome assessed was repetition of deliberate self-poisoning. The treatment group had 15.1% with one or more repeat episodes, while the control group had 17.3%; this difference was not statistically significant. The number of repeat episodes in the treatment group was about one half of that in the control group; this was statistically significant.

In summary, four studies of low-intensity post-suicide attempt interventions by phone or mail were identified. The results in the larger studies were either not statistically significant or were of modest efficacy.

Community-based Suicide Prevention Centers

Three observational studies about community-based suicide prevention centers were identified.

Walk[41] reported on a "Community Care" service implemented in Chichester, England, starting in 1958. The service was described as "with its blurred distinctions between in-patient, day-patient, out-patient and domiciliary treatment, its ready availability and its better contact with the community." (Unfortunately, no further details about the program were provided.) The suicide rate in five year periods before and after the program was started were compared. Their conclusion was "the introduction of Community Care may have protected some elderly patients from suicide, whereas it has had no clear effect on suicide among younger patients."

Bagley[42] examined data concerning the introduction of the Samaritan Suicide Prevention Schemes in 15 British towns. This program provides a suicide telephone hotline, available day or night. The hotline was staffed by clergy or lay workers who had undergone training designed to provide the workers with the skills to determine if the caller needed referral to clinical services. Each town in which the scheme was implemented was compared to a control town that matched on socioeconomic measures. The outcome assessed was the suicide rate in the same number of years before and after the program started, the actual number determined by the availability of data and ranged from 2 to 4 years. The average rate (per 100,000) for the treatment group towns was 13.03, decreasing to 12.27 after, and the average rate for the control towns was 12.56 before, increasing to 15.05 after. These changes were found to be statistically significant by a variety of measures.

Barraclough et al.[43] examined the same data using four different methods of choosing the control towns, including variations on the method of Bagley, matching on the pre-implementation suicide rate, or on the proportion of single-person households. They looked at suicide rates over three year pre- and post-implementation windows. They found no statistically significant difference in the suicide rates.

In summary, three studies of suicide-prevention centers were identified. One reported on an early, and very poorly described community-based program in England. Two examined the effect of the Samaritan Suicide Prevention Scheme in England and reached opposite conclusions. Overall the quality of these studies was low and the results inconclusive.

Hospital admission for attempted suicide

One RCT using hospital admission as the intervention for attempted suicide was identified.

Waterhouse and Platt[44] conducted their trial at the York District Hospital in England. Junior doctors were trained in the assessment of suicide attempts. Patients who presented to the ER and who were assessed as having no needs for immediate medical or psychiatric treatment were then randomized to either hospital admission or discharge to home. Those admitted to the hospital received no additional counseling or specific treatment. "Hospital admission consisted of little more than a bed, without further referral to other helping agencies." The median length of stay was 17 hours. The treatment group received the same instructions at discharge as the control group: to contact their general practitioners if the need for help arose. Thus, the treatment group differed from the control group only in the provision of hospital admission. For this pilot study the data were analyzed as if the junior doctor's initial assessment had been used, while the actual decision was made by the psychiatrist. The outcome assessed was repeated suicide attempts. In the first week post-discharge, two patients in each group had repeated attempts; at 16 weeks 3 patients in the treatment (admission) group had made repeated attempts, compared to 4 patients in the control group. The group sizes were not reported, so percentages can not be computed. No statistical measures were reported.

In summary, a single program studied the effect of brief hospital admission without additional treatment. Insufficient outcomes data were reported to determine its efficacy or statistical significance.

Other RCTs

Unutzer et al.[45] reported a multi-site trial in the US (including VA clinics in Texas) providing a collaborative care manager to primary care physicians to reduce suicidal ideation in depressed older patients. The depression care manager was a nurse or psychologist assigned to the primary care clinic; they assessed patients, educated patients about options for treating depression, and were in contact with the patients by phone or in-person every 2 weeks during the acute phase of treatment and monthly during the continuation phase continuing to 12 months. Patients in the control group and their primary care providers were informed that the patient met criteria for a depressive disorder; the patients could receive any of the available treatments, including antidepressants, counseling by the PCP, or referral for mental health care. Patients were randomly assigned to the treatment or the control groups. No completed suicides were reported in either group. The intended outcome measure reported for this trial was suicidal ideation, which did show statistically significant decreases at all follow up periods out to 24 months.

Mishara et al.[46] described a program implemented in Montreal in 2000-2002 to reduce suicidal behaviors in suicidal or depressed men by providing assistance to family or friends of those men who called a suicidal support center. Family or friends of the suicidal men were randomly assigned to one of four treatment interventions: (1) an information session that provided 2.5 hours of training in a group setting, (2) that information session plus phone follow up one week hence, (3) "rapid referral" for the suicidal man in which the family/friends had two in-person meetings with staff from the suicide center focusing on how to get the suicidal man into treatment with an appropriate agency, (4) telephone support counseling with flexible scheduling of follow up calls. The outcome assessed was suicide attempt. Results were not broken down by treatment group, and there was no control group providing treatment as usual, so the data were analyzed comparing post-intervention to pre-intervention. At study entry 22.9% of the participants reported a suicide attempt in the man in the previous 2 months; at 2 month follow up 10.6% reported an attempt in the previous 2 months, and at 6 month follow up 2.7% reported an attempt in the previous 2 months. Each of these differences was a statistically significant change. Participants also rated these programs as helpful to the men and the participants.

In summary, two other randomized, controlled trials were identified. The first, a high quality RCT, reported a collaborative care program in primary care clinics, and found no suicides in either the treatment or control groups. The second provided an intervention to the family or friends of men at high risk for suicide; the study was methodologically very weak and did not report the effect of treatments in comparison to a control group.

RESTRICTION OF ACCESS TO LETHAL MEANS

A large number of studies using observational data for restriction of access to lethal means were identified. These are grouped by means, first with firearms restriction, and then acetaminophen, and finally other toxicological agents.

Restriction of access to firearms

Twenty studies were identified concerning restriction of access to firearms. These are summarized in Evidence Table 3.

Restriction to access to firearms in the US

Loftin et al.[47] reported the effect of restrictive licensing of handguns in Washington, D.C., that began in 1976, and which "prohibited the purchase, sale, transfer, and possession of handguns by civilians," unless the firearm had been previously registered. They compared monthly suicide rates before and after the implementation of the law and found that the mean number of suicides per month declined from 2.6 to 2.0. This was statistically significant, both by a simple sampling model and also by an autoregressive integrated moving average (ARIMA) model commonly used in time-series modeling. To address the problem of secular changes, they studied non-gun-related suicides in the same region, and gun-related suicides in neighboring regions not subject to the law, and found no statistically significant decline in either measure over the same period. This handgun law was found to be unconstitutional by the US Supreme Court in June, 2008.

Ludwig and Cook[48] studied whether the introduction of the Brady Handgun Violence Prevention Act in the US, which instituted background checks and waiting periods, was associated with a reduction in suicide rates. Some states already met one or both of the requirements and served as controls; the authors also used regression modeling to control at the state level for alcohol consumption, and percentage of population in metropolitan areas, percentage below the poverty line, percentage African-American, and percentage in each of 7 age groups. They found that suicide rates had begun to fall before the introduction of the Brady Act; the Act was correlated with a reduction in suicides in victims 55 years or older, but only in states that changed both their waiting-period and background-check requirements.

Lott and Whitley[49] examined the effect of safe-storage gun laws in the US (which varied by state), and suicides in adolescents, including those in the age range of 15-19 years. Using data from the years 1979 to 1996, during which time 15 states adopted safe-storage laws (the year of enactment ranged from 1989 to 1996), they used weighted tobit regression models predicting the per capita suicide rate from a variety of fixed effect and control variables. The results showed a 5% decrease in gun suicides attributable to the safe-storage law; this was not statistically significant. A second set of more sophisticated regression models found: "… a couple of coefficients that indicated that gun suicides declined after the passage of the safe-storage law. However, in these cases, the evidence clearly rejects the hypothesis that the total number of suicides, committed by all methods, would be reduced."(p677). They did not provide the details supporting those results.

A similar study by Rosengart et al.[50] examined various kinds of handgun restriction laws in the US, using data from 1979 to 1998, and found that no law was statistically significantly associated with a change in the firearm suicide rate (in any age group). Webster et al.[51] examined related data from 1976 to 2001, for the age group of 18-20 years of the effects of minimum purchase age or child access prevention laws. They, found results that were either statistically insignificant or were of questionable causal believability for that age group.

Restriction of access to firearms in Canada

In Canada, a firearms control law was enforced starting in 1978 that required licensing, restricted certain sales, and increased criminal penalties for crimes involving firearms. The effects of this law have been examined in a number of studies, reported here chronologically.

Rich et al.[52] examined the law's effect in Toronto and Ontario. Mean rates in the five year periods before and after the law were compared; the data for the year 1978 were withheld because of the transition during the year. There was a small but not statistically significant decrease in the suicide rate for Toronto or for Ontario. They did find a statistically significant decrease in the fraction of suicides by shooting for men in Toronto, and a statistically significant increase in the fraction of men committing suicide by jumping. They considered this evidence of method substitution.

Carrington and Moyer[53] repeated the analysis of the data for Ontario studied by Rich et al.[52] using a slightly different data source, extended to include 1965-1977 and 1979-1989, and using age-standardized rates in a regression analysis. They found statistically significant increases in the firearm, non-firearm, and total suicide rates in the pre-legislation period, and decreases in those three rates (not significant for firearm suicide) in the post-legislation period. They considered their results as suggesting no method substitution.

Lester and Leenaars[54,55] looked at the law's effect for all of Canada for the 8 years prior (1969 to 1976) and eight years after (1978 to 1985). Examination of the raw statistics showed that the rate of suicide by firearm and fraction of suicide by firearm had a statistically significant decrease, but that both the overall suicide rate and the suicide rate by other means increased. A post-hoc linear regression analysis showed that before the law, the rates for suicide by firearm and by other methods, along with the fraction of suicides by firearm were all increasing, while after the law was enforced, these quantities were all decreasing (although the suicide rate by other methods was not statistically significant). They concluded that there was not evidence for method substitution.

Leenaars and Lester[56] examined the same data separately for men and women. For men, the firearms suicide rate and the rate for other methods both increased in the post-legislation period, while the fraction of men using firearms for suicide decreased. They considered this is as evidence of switching in men. For women, the rates were stable or declined, and there was no evidence for switching.

Lester[57] reanalyzed the Canadian data using two alternative measure of firearms availability: accidental death rate from firearms, and average of fraction of suicides and homicides committed by firearm. These data were available for 1970 to 1995. One or both of these measures was statistically significantly correlated with the firearm suicide rate (positively) and both the total suicide rate and the suicide rate by other methods (negatively). Lester also found a negative time trend for the firearm suicide rate, and a positive time trend for the suicide rate by other methods.

Lester concluded that these data were consistent with method substitution.

Leenaars and Lester[58] reexamined the Canadian data to determine the effect of the legislation on suicide rates by age group. The post-legislation mean handgun suicide rates declined for ages 35-44, 45-54, and 55-64 (all statistically significantly), and increased for ages 15-24, 25-34, 65-74, and 75+ (the increases for 25-34 and 65-74 were not statistically significant). They concluded that there was little evidence for the effectiveness of the act in reducing suicide for those 65 and up.

Leenaars et al.[59], looked at the same data using regression modeling. The firearm suicide rate showed an increasing trend before the legislation, no step-effect at the time of the legislation, and a negative slope for the interaction term, indicating a declining trend after the legislation. The same pattern was seen in the data for men only, but for women the pre-legislation trend was not significant and the post-legislation decline was statistically significant but small in magnitude. The results also suggested a displacement effect for men, but not for women. The authors also conducted a multivariate regression including a variety of social indicators, such as income, and birth, marriage, and divorce rates as predictor variables. This showed a statistically significant decrease in firearm suicide rates for both men and women, and evidence for switching in men.

Bridges[60] used a similar approach to examine the effect of a different Canadian law passed in 1991 that mandated additional pre-purchase screening and a 28-day waiting period over 7 years periods before and after the introduction of the law. The mean rate for firearm suicide and the fraction of suicide by firearm decreased, while the total suicide rate increased. Trends were checked by using separate linear regressions in the pre- and post-legislation periods. The total suicide rate, the firearms suicide rate, the rate for other methods, and the fraction of suicides by firearm all had negative slopes in the pre-legislation period; in the post-legislation period there were negative (but small) slopes for the firearms suicide rate and the fraction of suicide by firearms. There was no evidence for switching.

Cheung and Dewa[61] examined the effect of the same Canadian 1991 law on the suicide rate in adolescents ages 15-19. Using a time-series model over the years 1979-1999, they found a decrease in the firearms suicide rate after 1991, but a corresponding increase in the rate of hanging, consistent with method switching.

Restriction to access to firearms in Australia/New Zealand

Snowdon and Harris[62] looked at the firearm suicide rate in Australia's five largest states, one of which (South Australia) enacted a stringent firearm examination and licensing law in 1980. The suicide rates were examined over the years 1968 to 1989. The rate in South Australia was statistically significantly lower when compared to the four other states, and when compared directly with the state of Victoria, the most similar state on demographic measures. The decrease in South Australia was accompanied by an increase in suicide by other means. They were unable to reach firm conclusions about method substitution.

Chapman et al.[63] studied whether Australia's firearms restrictions, which were enacted in 1996 and included prohibitions on private ownership of semi-automatic and pump-action rifles and shotguns, and also a buy-back program of existing firearms, were associated with a reduction in suicide rates. The data were analyzed using a negative binomial model. The authors reported that the firearm suicide rate, which was already decreasing at 3% per year, further dropped to 7.4% per year after the law change. The total suicide rate changed from a 2.3% increase per year to a 4.1% decrease, although at the time of the law change, the total rate did transiently increase in absolute numbers.

Cantor and Slater[64] examined the effect of firearm control legislation in the state of Queensland requiring a 28 day waiting period and a safety test which came into effect in 1992 on the suicide rate in metropolitan, provincial, and rural areas in that state. The mean annual suicide rate per 100,000 in the two years before the change was compared to the rate in the two years following the change. There were statistically significant decreases in the firearms suicide rate in the metropolitan (3.6 to 2.3) and provincial (5.2 to 3.1) but not in the rural areas (7.2 to 8.2, non-significant). A subgroup analysis showed that the significant decreases were in men age 15-29 in the metropolitan and provincial areas. There were statistically significant increases by men in metropolitan and provincial areas in the use drug overdose and hanging, although the total rate for men decreased slightly.

Ozanne-Smith et al.[65] studied the effect of firearm regulation in Australia, introduced first in the state of Victoria, and then several years later in the rest of Australia. The legislation banned certain classes of firearms, required registration and a safety class, and included a 1 year longarms buyback scheme. They used a Poisson regression model with data over three periods: 1979-86 (no legislation), 1988-1995 (legislation introduced in Victoria), and 1997-2000 (similar legislation introduced in rest of Australia). The suicide rates in Victoria declined in each successive period at a statistically significant rate (a 72% decline in the average annual frequency from the first to the third period). They did not report on data directly relevant to the problems of displacement or method substitution.

Beautrais et al.[66] reported on reduction of suicide rates in New Zealand associated with restrictive firearms legislation, enacted in 1992, and which mandated police assessment, testing, and licensing of gun owners, along with strict requirements for gun security and storage. Their analysis used a variety of regression models, including Poisson regression, a time-series forecasting model, a polynomial model, and an auto-regressive model, over three intervals: before the implementation, the four-year period of implementation (1993-96), and after the implementation period. They reported a decline in the suicide rate for youth (15-24y), adult (25+y), and combined populations over time; this trend was most marked for youth suicide. A similar pattern was seen for firearm suicide as a percentage of total suicides. Use of various models showed no evidence for a decline in the overall rate of suicide.

In summary, a large number of studies concerning restricting access to firearms were identified. A number of the studies reported variations on analyses of the same or very similar data sets. All compared the suicide rates before and after the implementation of laws restricting access to firearms. Methodological issues common to the analysis of observational data were present, especially addressing statistical fluctuations by using longer windows for the pre- or post-intervention periods, while trying to minimize the effect of other, unmeasured, socioeconomic trends, such as changes in the divorce or unemployment rate. The results as reported are mixed, but suggest some protective effect at least in some groups as determined by age and gender. The question of possible shifts to other methods leading to no net reduction in suicide (method substitution) remains unresolved.

Restriction of access to acetaminophen (UK: paracetamol, US Brand: Tylenol, others)

The UK enacted legislation in September 1998 that limited the package size of paracetamol and salicylates (including aspirin). Paracetamol is commonly used in suicide by overdose and if untreated can cause fatal liver failure. The effect of this legislation has been reported in a number of studies, presented here chronologically.

Prince et al.[67] reported on the number of patients referred to a tertiary care liver unit at a single hospital, and the number of national liver transplantation requests from September 1995 to August 1999. Monthly rates for both declined after the legislation, in spite of a preexisting increasing trend in national transplant referrals.

Turvill et al.[68] reported on the number of paracetamol overdoses at one London hospital from September 1995 to August 1999. The number of overdoses declined by 21% (with a 64% decline in severe overdoses, as determined by existing guidelines) after the legislation. There was no change in the rate of benzodiazepine overdoses, which served as a control measure.

Robinson et al.[69] measured the several parameters before the legislation (January through June 1998) and after (same months, 1999) in patients at a hospital in Belfast. They found statistically significant decreases in the estimated quantity of paracetamol ingested, the serum paracetamol concentration, the percentage of patients admitted to the hospital, the percentage of patients given antidote, a measure of liver function (INR) and concentrations of liver enzymes.

Steen et al.[70] examined the effect of the legislation on paracetamol-related deaths in Scotland. They compared all paracetamol-related deaths in the years 1996-1997 and the years 1999-2000. The rate for the two years preceding the year of implementation was 1.93 per 100,000; the rate for the latter two years was 1.78 per 100,000. This change was not significant by the chi-square test. Informally, they observed a declining trend in the paracetamol-only deaths in males before the legislation, which reversed in the year 2000. They also noted that Scotland has a markedly higher suicide rate than England or Wales.

Hughes et al.[71] counted the number of admissions to a Birmingham, UK hospital or a related hospital's liver unit as the result of paracetamol poisonings for three years before and three years after 1998. Hospital admissions showed a 31% reduction, and liver unit admissions showed a 50% reduction. No statistical analysis was conducted.

Hawton et al.[72] and Hawton[73] compared the suicide deaths in the two years before the change with the deaths in the year after the change. There were statistically significant reductions in deaths for both classes of compounds considered individually, but not when taken with other drugs or taken together. They also found that the number of admissions to hospital liver units and the number of liver transplantations declined over the same intervals. The number of non-fatal self-poisonings with paracematol or salicylates declined in absolute numbers, comparing the previous year to the subsequent year, but there was no decline the proportion of total cases of self-poisoning. They concluded that "legislation restricting pack sizes of paracetamol and salicylates in the United Kingdom has had substantial beneficial effects on mortality and morbidity associated with self-poisoning using these drugs."

Hawton et al.[74] repeated the above analysis, adding another post-legislation year, and also included trend modeling with data from 1993 to 2002 to test for step change at the time of the legislation. They found a 29% decrease in paracetamol-related deaths, and 46% decrease in salicyclate-related deaths. They also evidence for a downward step change for both paracetamol and salicyclate overdoses at the time of the legislation. Liver unit admissions, liver transplants, and nonfatal paracetamol and aspirin overdoses decreased after the legislation.

Morgan et al.[75] analyzed UK national data for the package restriction using chi-square (and later analyzed the same data using segmented linear regression: Morgan et al.[76]). To control for secular trends, they compared the paracetamol deaths to those from paracetamol in combination with other compounds, aspirin (which was also limited by the same legislation), antidepressants, and non-drug poisoning suicides. There were declines (negative slopes) in age-standardized mortality rates for all the groups studied. There was a downward step change in those rates for paracetamol poisoning, with a similar step change for aspirin and antidepressants, but not for paracetamol compounds or non-drug poisoning suicides. Thus, while the paracetamol deaths declined, other suicide deaths also declined over the same period. They conclude that there is "little evidence" to associate the reduction in paracetamol-related suicides with the package size reductions.

Similar restrictions in Ireland were introduced starting in October 1997. An abstract by Donohoe and Tracey[77] reported no statistically significant difference in the number of overdose cases reported to the National Poisons Information Centre in Dublin in 1998, compared to 1997. There was a slight but not statistically significant decline in severe overdoses.

For Australia, Balit et al.[78] reported on the effect of a recall of paracetamol-containing products during two periods in 2000 in response to threatened insertion of poisons into those products. The outcome measures were the number of calls to a poison information center and the number of admissions to a toxicology inpatient service, both in New South Wales. These measures during the recall periods were compared with corresponding measures in the same months of the three preceding years (1997-1999). At one site, there was no statistically significant change in the percentage of calls for paracetamol or aspirin, but an increase for ibuprofen; at the other site, there was no statistically significant change in the presentations for paracetamol or ibuprofen, but an increase for aspirin. They concluded that there was no reduction in deliberate self-poisonings during a period of restricted availability.

In summary, a number of studies of the effect of UK restrictions on paracetamol showed declines in suicides coincident with those restrictions. However, there is some evidence from time-series modeling that this was part of a longer downward trend in suicide. Many of the studies had very short post-intervention periods. A small of number of studies in other countries reported equivocal results. Unlike the area of restriction of access to firearms, there was little analysis of method substitution.

Restriction of access to respiratory toxins

Kreitman[79] studied deaths due to asphyxiation by "domestic gas" in the UK (England, Wales, Scotland) in relationship to changes in the production of such gas from coal to natural gas that significantly lowered the carbon monoxide content over approximately a decade starting in the late 1950s. Kreitman reported that the reduction in carbon monoxide content was paralleled by a drop in carbon monoxide poisoning deaths during that same interval; this was found in both sexes and all age groups. The decline was significant enough to overcome an increase in the other rates of suicide for both young men and women to produce a net overall decline.

Kendell[80] reported data on the effect in Scotland of the UK regulation requiring all cars sold after December 31, 1992 to have catalytic converters, thereby decreasing the carbon monoxide content of the exhaust gas. For men, the fraction of all suicides attributed to poisoning by gases other than domestic gas showed a statistically significant decline (chi-square for trend), with a smaller but also statistically significant decline for women. A data over a somewhat shorter interval in England and Wales showed the same pattern.

Amos et al.[81] studied deaths due to carbon monoxide poisoning by car exhaust in England and Wales for the years before (1987-1992) and after (1993-1998) European legislation requiring that all new car have catalytic converters. For all age groups and both sexes there was a decline in deaths from car exhaust, and in the percentage of all suicides that were due to car exhaust. These comparisons were made using the raw statistics, not age/population adjusted numbers. They also performed a hierarchical multiple linear regression that included an interaction term that was the product of the two study periods; however, they reported only the statistical tests on the regression analysis, not the coefficients. They noted that the decline in car exhaust asphyxiations had started, at least in some groups, prior to the implementation of the law.

Routley[82] conducted a similar study in Australia, where 1986 regulations added catalytic converters to new cars. Using data from 1971 to 1995, they found that motor vehicle exhaust gas suicide rates increased generally increased over time, even after the regulation. Numbers of patients hospitalized for motor vehicle exhaust gas suicide attempts also increased during the interval. A sample of 100 cases of exhaust gas suicide in the state of Victoria were reviewed. The fraction of vehicles used in these suicides manufactured after 1986 was not significantly different from the fraction for the Victorian motor fleet at large. They concluded that catalytic converters were not associated with a decline in motor vehicle exhaust suicide number, rate, or proportion.

In summary, four studies were found concerning restricting access to respiratory agents. One study found that changing the source of domestic gas in the UK resulted in a decrease in carbon monoxide poisonings. The effect of catalytic converters on car exhaust asphyxiation reported in three studies was mixed.

Access to/effect of pharmacologic agents

Oliver and Hetzel[83] reported on the relationship between changes in the availability of sedative drugs due to subsidization of health care in Australia in 1960, which increased the availability and a subsequent reduction in 1967 of the amounts provided in each prescription, and the effect on the national suicide rate over the same time period. They found an increase in the incidence of barbiturate deaths in adults during the time of increased availability, and a subsequent decrease with the limitation on sedative amounts.

Whitlock[84] conducted a similar study in Brisbane, Australia, for the years 1962 to 1973, and found a similar result: that barbiturate suicide deaths tracked their increase and then decrease in availability. This effect was more prominent in women, for whom barbiturate overdose was more common. There was already an increasing trend in suicide rates before the increase associated with the availability of barbiturates. Whitlock also addressed the changing use of other medications, such as benzodiazepines and antidepressants, which might have substituted for barbiturates, either therapeutically or as methods of self-poisoning, but the fact that the changes in use extended over multi-year periods, and the lack of a single intervention greatly complicates the analysis of this observational data, and the detection of method substitution and secular trends. Whitlock did note that there had been no deaths from carbon monoxide poisoning in those aged 65 and older after 1967, when domestic gas was switched to a nontoxic source.

In summary, two studies in Australia on the effect of access to sedative drugs lethal in overdose showed a decline in the suicide rate that tracked restrictions on their availability.

Bridge barriers

One study on the effect of bridge barriers in reducing suicide by jumping was identified.

Beautrais[85] reported on the effect of removing existing screens from a bridge in an "Australasian metropolitan area." The location was described in a disguised fashion so as to avoid attracting further attention to it. Existing screens were removed by the action of the city council in 1995 because they were felt to actually impede access to rescuing suicide attempters and for aesthetic reasons. Suicide rates by jumping at that bridge and other bridges were compared in three-year periods before and after the barrier removal. The rate (per 100,000) at the bridge before the barriers were removed was 0.29; this increased to 1.29 after the removal. The number of suicides at the other bridges declined after the barrier removal, and the citywide total before and after remained constant. Beautrais presented additional data on the subject's mental health diagnosis (mostly, schizophrenia) suggesting that the act of barrier removal increased the suicide rate for mental patients because of its location near the regions largest inpatient psychiatric facility, and that the removal did not merely shift suicides from other bridges.

In summary, a single observational study reported an increase in suicide by jumping after protective screens were removed from a bridge; there was some evidence that the removal led to an actual increase in suicide, not merely displacement from other bridges.

Restriction on Media Reporting of Suicides

One controlled study reported on media restriction of reporting of suicides.

Motto[86] examined the suicide rate in Detroit during a 268-day period in 1967-8 when a newspaper strike lead to the complete cessation of publication. The suicide rate of the blackout period was compared to the average rate during the same days in the previous four years. The rate for men was the same (16.7 per 100,000), while the rate for women dropped from 7.6 to 3.0; the decline was statistically significant. An overall declining trend starting before the blackout period was noted.

In summary, a single observational study on media restriction during an extended newspaper strike showed a decline in suicides for women, and no change for men. There may have been an preexisting declining trend in suicide starting before the strike.

KEY QUESTION #3: What evidence is still needed to establish various strategies as the most promising (framed as research questions to guide and focus continued research to expand knowledge regarding the effectiveness of suicide prevention approaches)?

Multifaceted interventions are supported by consistent evidence, although of very mixed quality. Even if such programs are later determined to be robustly successful, the question of which components in those programs are causally related to the reduction in suicides has not been addressed. This sets as a research issue determining which components work best in which combinations for which populations. The issue of whether some sets of components may have facilitative or synergistic effects has not been addressed.

Psychosocial intervention for suicide attempters have considerable face validity as they address a group with manifest evidence of suicide risk, but there is no consistent evidence in their support in spite of a moderate number of randomized controlled trials that been conducted. This is an area of obvious and considerable interest to the VA, which is now using similar approaches in its clinical programs to identify and track those at high risk with suicide risk flags, screening tools, and suicide prevention coordinators. An additional factor that seems relevant but rarely directly studied is the effect of forming a consistent relationship with a single provider, a therapeutic alliance, and its role in providing a protective degree of social connection, and reducing the harmful consequences of social isolation.

Further randomized controlled trials and high-quality observational studies are definitely needed. Without waiting for such to be completed, and independent of which program components the VA decides to pursue, there are two supporting initiatives that could be implemented in parallel. The first concerns standardizing vocabulary, and the second concerns electronic medical records.

First, all suicide prevention programs are dependent on the accuracy with which assessments of suicidality are conducted. The term "suicide attempt" covers a very broad array of self-injurious behaviors, from intentionally planned, high lethality events that were interrupted by mere happenstance, through low lethality acts marked by a small risk of physical harm, impulsivity, and a high likelihood of discovery by others. Others have noted the importance of establishing and using a consistent nomenclature in this area.

A very important reason for accurately describing the severity of suicide attempts is that an attempt is widely recognized as a significant risk factor for completions. Although most completed suicides are first attempts[2] and attempters vary in important ways from completers,[3] it is known that survivors of highly lethal attempts have similar clinical and psychosocial profiles to antemorten profiles of suicide completers. This suggests that subcategorization of attempt by lethality (or perhaps other factors) may be clinically useful.

Second, because the VA uses a single, integrated computerized medical record system for all of its clinical activities, any improvements in vocabulary along with new screening and tracking tools would allow for data gathering as part of routine practice – especially for establishing patterns and risk factors for suicide attempts – in advance of formally conducted observational studies or controlled trials.

SUMMARY AND DISCUSSION

In this chapter, we describe the limitations of our review and then present our conclusions. We also discuss the implications of our findings for future research.

LIMITATIONS

PUBLICATION BIAS
Our literature search procedures were extensive. It was not possible to conduct formal tests for publication bias, but even with such tests it is not possible to exclude the possibility that such bias exists. Therefore, readers are cautioned about this possibility.

STUDY QUALITY
An important limitation common to systematic reviews is the quality of the original studies. Recent attempts to define elements of study design and execution that are related to bias have shown that in many cases, such efforts are not reproducible and do not distinguish study results based on bias. Therefore, the current approach is to avoid rejecting studies or using quality criteria to adjust the results of the review. We did use the Delphi list criteria as a descriptive measure of quality.[11] As there is a lack of empirical evidence regarding study characteristics and their relationship to bias, we did not attempt to use other criteria. Other aspects of the design and execution of a trial may be related to bias, but we do not yet have good measures of these elements. Because of the small number of studies found, it was not possible to do sensitivity analyses based on study quality.

HETEROGENEITY
Clearly, the populations being assessed were different, and there were also important differences in how some key variables were measured, characteristics of the interventions, and outcomes measured, among others. This heterogeneity further limits our ability to draw strong conclusions.

APPLICABILITY OF FINDINGS
Green & Glasgow[87] provide a framework for evaluating the relevance, generalization, and applicability of research. Their framework includes assessing the participation rate, the intended target population, the representativeness of the setting, the representativeness of the individuals, and evaluating information about implementation and assessment of outcomes. As these data are rarely reported in the studies we reviewed, conclusions about applicability are necessarily weak.

COMPARISON WITH SYSTEMATIC REVIEWS AND META-ANALYSES

We now discuss how our results relate to those published in other, similar systematic reviews and meta-analyses.

Gaynes et al.[7] presented a systematic review for the US Preventive Services Task Force on screening for suicide risk in adults with a focus on primary care settings. They found "extremely limited" evidence that could be used for assessment and management of the risk of suicide by primary care clinicians. "No studies address the overarching question of whether screening for suicide risk in primary care patients improves outcome…. Regarding whether interventions for those at risk reduce suicide attempts or completions, the poor generalizability of the studies makes the overall strength of evidence fair, at best, while the results are mixed. Although some trends suggest incremental benefit from several interventions, no consistent statistically significant effects have emerged for interventions for which more than 1 study has been done."

Mann et al.[1] whose conceptual model and results guided the construction of our review, concluded that "the most promising interventions are physician education, means restriction, and gatekeeper education." However their conclusion about physician education was based on studies in countries (Hungary, Japan, and the island of Gotland, Sweden) whose suicide rates and patterns are not similar to those in the US population. The gatekeeper education result followed from a single study, the multifaceted USAF suicide prevention program, which actually provided significantly more services than just gatekeeping.

Morgan and Majeed[88] reviewed the UK studies on paracetamol restriction, and found some evidence for a decrease in admission to liver units and transplant requests after the introduction of the restrictions. However, they noted as complicating factors small sample sizes, the lack of a precise definition of paracetamol poisoning, and the absence of any control groups in the studies examined. They also observed that in spite of the restrictions, paracetamol was still commonly used as a means of suicide.

Hawton et al.[89] conducted a review for the Cochrane Collaboration on psychosocial and pharmacological treatments for deliberate self-harm. They found non-significant trends for problem-solving therapy, provision of an emergency contact card, intensive aftercare plus outreach, and antidepressant treatment. They concluded that "considerable uncertainty" remained, and that the clinical trials reviewed to date had been too small.

Crawford et al.[90] reported a systematic review of RCTs for psychosocial interventions following episodes of self-harm, and for 18 studies found no difference in the suicide rate between treatment and control groups. Three of the studies involved children or adolescents. Crawford et al. also included psychotherapeutic interventions – none of which were included in our review. Sample size and lack of statistical power were identified as complicating factors. They argued for pursuing public health approaches, such as means restriction and media guidelines for reporting.

Other non-systematic reviews

One non-systematic review relevant to our report was identified. Lester[91] reviewed the evidence supporting the use of suicide prevention centers. Fourteen independent studies were identified, of which seven showed evidence for protective effects, but these were not consistent across gender, age groups, and suicide methods. When protective effects were found, they were often small in magnitude. Lester combined the studies using a meta-analysis, which did achieve statistical significance, with a correlation coefficient of -0.16 (which is equivalent to an effect size of -0.32).

Reviews of mental health interventions

Our review did not focus on purely mental health interventions. These have been the subject of other reviews. Perhaps somewhat surprisingly given the role of depressive disorders as significant risk factors for suicide, the evidence in support of the use of antidepressants is rather weak. Isaacson and Rich[92] in nonsystematic review on the protective effects of antidepressants for suicide concluded, in part, "Pooled data from controlled clinical trials of antidepressants have not demonstrated a suicide preventive effect, but patient selection and the brief time of most trials limits the power of the data. Some reports from either long-term or very large databases have provided evidence that antidepressants prevent suicide."(p153)

Some of the best evidence for psychopharmacologic interventions that reduce suicide risk is for lithium in the treatment of bipolar disorder. Baldessarini et al.[93] reported a meta-analysis of 31 published studies that showed a robust protective effect of lithium for both completed and attempted suicides for both bipolar disorder and other mood disorders. There is also some evidence supporting the use of the antipsychotic clozapine to reduce suicide attempts in schizophrenia. Further details appear in a non-systematic review by Hennen and Baldessarini[94] and a systematic review by Aguilar and Siris.[95]

CONCLUSIONS

With the above limitations in mind, we reached the conclusions displayed below.

KEY QUESTION #1: What are the new or improved suicide prevention strategies (e.g., hotlines, outreach programs, peer counseling, treatment coordination programs, and new counseling approaches) that show promise for Veterans?

KEY QUESTION #2: What solid evidence base supports the most promising strategies?

Multicomponent interventions in military personnel probably reduce the risk of suicide. The largest and best described such study is by Knox, and this article provides the most convincing evidence of effectiveness. The report of success of a program in Yugoslavia modeled after the Knox program increases our confidence that the effect is real. A similar program was developed for the US Navy and Marine Corps. However, as with any multicomponent intervention shown to be successful, there are still numerous questions about the relative merit of inclusion of each individual component (could the same effect be achieved with fewer components?) or the possible increase in effectiveness of adding other components, and optimizing the effectiveness of each additional component. Additionally, there are no data about its effect in non-military populations, although veterans would seem to be sufficiently close to a military population that some transferability of results could be assumed. (GRADE quality of evidence = Low, meaning further research is very likely to have an important impact on our confidence in the estimate of effect and is likely to change the estimate)

There are insufficient studies of suicide prevention programs specifically in veterans to draw conclusions (GRADE quality of evidence = Very Low, meaning any estimate of effect is uncertain)

Psychosocial interventions following a suicide attempt are, at the very best, only minimally effective (GRADE quality of evidence = Moderate, meaning further research is likely to have an important impact on our confidence in the estimate of the effect and may change the estimate).

There are insufficient data to reach conclusions about Community-based Suicide Prevention Centers (GRADE quality of evidence = Very Low , meaning any estimate of effect is uncertain)

We found no studies that assessed the specific effectiveness of any of hotlines, outreach programs as primary prevention interventions, peer counseling, treatment coordination programs, and new counseling programs.

Restriction of access to lethal means probably has an effect on cause-specific suicides, although its effect on total suicides is less clear (GRADE quality of evidence = Low, meaning further research is very likely to have an important impact on our confidence in the estimate of effect and is likely to change the estimate)

KEY QUESTION #3: What evidence is still needed to establish various strategies as the most promising (framed as research questions to guide and focus continued research to expand knowledge regarding the effectiveness of suicide prevention approaches)?

Multifaceted interventions are supported by consistent evidence, although of very mixed quality. Even if such programs are later determined to be robustly successful, the question of which components in those programs are causally related to the reduction in suicides has not been addressed. This sets as a research issue determining which components work best in which combinations for which populations. The issue of whether some sets of components may have facilitative or synergistic effects has not been addressed.

Psychosocial intervention for suicide attempters have considerable face validity as they address a group with manifest evidence of suicide risk, but there is no consistent evidence in their support in spite of a moderate number of randomized controlled trials that been conducted. This is an area of obvious and considerable interest to the VA, which is now using similar approaches in its clinical programs to identify and track those at high risk with suicide risk flags, screening tools, and suicide prevention coordinators. An additional factor that seems relevant but rarely directly studied is the effect of forming a consistent relationship with a single provider, a therapeutic alliance, and its role in providing a protective degree of social connection, and reducing the harmful consequences of social isolation.

Further randomized controlled trials and high-quality observational studies are definitely needed. Without waiting for such to be completed, and independent of which program components the

41

VA decides to pursue, there are two supporting initiatives that could be implemented in parallel. The first concerns standardizing vocabulary, and the second concerns electronic medical records.

First, all suicide prevention programs are dependent on the accuracy with which assessments of suicidality are conducted. The term "suicide attempt" covers a very broad array of self-injurious behaviors, from intentionally planned, high lethality events that were interrupted by mere happenstance, through low lethality acts marked by a small risk of physical harm, impulsivity, and a high likelihood of discovery by others. Others have noted the importance of establishing and using a consistent nomenclature in this area.[96] It is critical for further advances in suicide reduction that such attempts are carried through.

A very important reason for accurately describing the severity of suicide attempts is that an attempt is widely recognized as a significant risk factor for completions. Although most completed suicides are first attempts[2] and attempters vary in important ways from completers,[3] it is known that survivors of highly lethal attempts have similar clinical and psychosocial profiles to antemorten profiles of suicide completers. This suggests that subcategorization of attempt by lethality (or perhaps other factors) may be clinically useful.

Completed suicides are thought to be more easily determined, as they are judged such on the basis of a coroner or medical examiner ruling. In most cases the determination is straightforward, but others, such as single-occupant car crashes, raise the issue of disguised suicides, where intent may have been willfully hidden for reasons of shame or insurance coverage. Crawford et al.[90] noted difficulties in using reported suicides because of problems of ascertainment. Addressing these forensic issues is mostly outside the purview of the VA.

Second, because the VA uses a single, integrated computerized medical record system for all of its clinical activities, any improvements in vocabulary along with new screening and tracking tools would allow for data gathering as part of routine practice – especially for establishing patterns and risk factors for suicide attempts – in advance of formally conducted observational studies or controlled trials.

REFERENCES

1.   Mann JJ, Apter A, Bertolote J, Beautrais A, Currier D, Haas A, et al. Suicide prevention strategies: a systematic review. JAMA 2005; 294:2064-74.

2.   Mann JJ. A current perspective of suicide and attempted suicide. Ann Intern Med 2002; 136:302-11.

3.   Paris J. Predicting and preventing suicide: do we know enough to do either? Harv Rev Psychiatry 2006; 14:233-40.

4.   Hankin CS, Spiro A 3rd, Miller DR, Kazis L. Mental disorders and mental health treatment among U.S. Department of Veterans Affairs outpatients: the Veterans Health Study. Am J Psychiatry 1999; 156:1924-30.

5.   Zivin K, Kim HM, McCarthy JF, Austin KL, Hoggatt KJ, Walters H, et al. Suicide mortality among individuals receiving treatment for depression in the Veterans Affairs health system: associations with patient and treatment setting characteristics. Am J Public Health 2007; 97:(12)2193-8. Serious Mental Illness Treatment Research and Evaluation Center (SMITREC), Health Services Research and Development (HSR&D) Center of Excellence, Department of Veterans Affairs, Ann Arbor, Mich, USA. kzivin@umich.edu.

6.   Milliken CS, Auchterlonie JL, Hoge CW. Longitudinal assessment of mental health problems among active and reserve component soldiers returning from the Iraq war. JAMA 2007; 298:2141-8.

7.   Gaynes BN, West SL, Ford CA, Frame P, Klein J, Lohr KN. Screening for suicide risk in adults: a summary of the evidence for the U.S. Preventive Services Task Force. Ann Intern Med 2004; 140:822-35.

8.   Pirkis J, Blood RW, Beautrais A, Burgess P, Skehans J. Media guidelines on the reporting of suicide. Crisis 2006; 27:82-7.

9.   Oxman AD, Guyatt GH. Validation of an index of the quality of review articles. J Clin Epidemiol 1991; 44:1271-8.

10.   Shea BJ, Grimshaw JM, Wells GA, Boers M, Andersson N, Hamel C, et al. Development of AMSTAR: a measurement tool to assess the methodological quality of systematic reviews. BMC Med Res Methodol 2007; 7:10

11.   Verhagen AP, de Vet HC, de Bie RA, Kessels AG, Boers M, Bouter LM, et al. The Delphi list: a criteria list for quality assessment of randomized clinical trials for conducting systematic reviews developed by Delphi consensus. J Clin Epidemiol 1998; 51:1235-41.

12.   Atkins D, Best D, Briss PA, Eccles M, Falck-Ytter Y, Flottorp S, et al. Grading quality of evidence and strength of recommendations. BMJ 2004; 328:1490

13.   James LC, Kowalski TJ. Suicide prevention in an army infantry division: a multi-disciplinary program. Mil Med 1996; 161:97-101.

14. McDaniel WW, Rock M, Grigg JR. Suicide prevention at a United States Navy training command. Mil Med 1990; 155:173-5.

15. Knox KL, Litts DA, Talcott GW, Feig JC, Caine ED. Risk of suicide and related adverse outcomes after exposure to a suicide prevention programme in the US Air Force: cohort study. BMJ 2003; 327:1376

16. Jones DE, Kenedy KR, Hawkes C, Hourani LA, Long MA, Robbins D. Suicide prevention in Navy and Marine Corps: applying the public health model. Navy Med 2001; 92:31-6.

17. Kennedy CH, Cook JH, Poole DR, Brunson CL, Jones DE. Review of the first year of an overseas military gambling treatment program. Mil Med 2005; 170:(8)683-7. Substance Abuse Rehabilitation Program, United States Naval Hospital, Okinawa, Japan.

18. Rozanov VA, Mokhovikov AN, Stiliha R. Successful model of suicide prevention in the Ukraine military environment. Crisis 2002; 23:171-7.

19. Dedic G, Panic M. Suicide prevention program in the Army of Serbia and Montenegro. Mil Med 2007; 172:(5)551-5. Department for Mental Health, Military Medical Academy, 11000 Belgrade, Crno- travska 17, Serbia.

20. Robinson J, McGorry P, Harris MG, Pirkis J, Burgess P, Hickie I, et al. Australia's National Suicide Prevention Strategy: the next chapter. Aust Health Rev 2006; 30:(3)271-6. ORYGEN Research Centre, University of Melbourne, 35 Poplar Road, Parkville, Melbourne, VIC 3052, Australia. jo.robinson@mh.org.au.

21. National Suicide Prevention Strategy for England. National Institute for Mental Health in England, Care Services Improvement Partnership.

22. Koons CR, Robins CJ, Tweed JL, Lynch TR. Efficacy of dialectical behavior therapy in women veterans with borderline personality disorder. Behavior Therapy 2001; 32:371-90.

23. Ilgen MA, Jain A, Lucas E, Moos RH. Substance use-disorder treatment and a decline in attempted suicide during and after treatment. J Stud Alcohol Drugs 2007; 68:(4)503-9. Center for Health Care Evaluation, Department of Veterans Affairs Palo Alto Health Care System, 795 Willow Road (MPD 152), Menlo Park, California 94025, USA. Mark. Ilgen@va.gov.

24. Gibbons RD, Brown CH, Hur K, Marcus SM, Bhaumik DK, Mann JJ . Relationship between antidepressants and suicide attempts: an analysis of the Veterans Health Administration data sets. Am J Psychiatry 2007; 164:(7)1044-9. Center for Health Statistics, University of Illinois at Chicago, Chicago, IL 60614, USA. rdgib@uic.edu.

25. Welu TC. A follow-up program for suicide attempters: evaluation of effectiveness. Suicide Life Threat Behav 1977; 7:17-20.

26. Ternansen PE, Bywater C. S.A.F.E.R.: A follow-up service for attempted suicide in Vancover. Canadian Psychiatric Association Journal 1975; 20:29-34.

27. Allard R, Marshall M, Plante MC. Intensive follow-up does not decrease the risk of repeat suicide attempts. Suicide Life Threat Behav 1992; 22:303-14.

28. Chowdury N, Hicks RC, Kreitman N. Evaluation of an after-care service for parasuicide (attempted suicide) patients. Social Psychiatry 1973; 8:67-81.

29. Gardner R, Hanka R, O'Brien VC, Page AJ, Rees R. Psychological and social evaluation in cases of deliberate self-poisoning admitted to a general hospital. Br Med J 1977; 2:1567-70.

30. Gibbons JS, Butler J, Urwin P, Gibbons JL. Evaluation of a social work service for self-poisoning patients. Br J Psychiatry 1978; 133:111-8.

31. Hawton K, Bancroft J, Catalan J, Kingston B, Stedeford A, Welch N. Domiciliary and out-patient treatment of self-poisoning patients by medical and non-medical staff. Psychol Med 1981; 11:169-77.

32. Hawton K, McKeown S, Day A, Martin P, O'Connor M, Yule J. Evaluation of out-patient counselling compared with general practitioner care following overdoses. Psychol Med 1987; 17:751-61.

33. Guthrie E, Kapur N, Mackway-Jones K, Chew-Graham C, Moorey J, Mendel E, et al. Randomised controlled trial of brief psychological intervention after deliberate self poisoning. BMJ 2001; 323:135-8.

34. Bennewith O, Stocks N, Gunnell D, Peters TJ, Evans MO, Sharp DJ. General practice based intervention to prevent repeat episodes of deliberate self harm: cluster randomised controlled trial. BMJ 2002; 324:1254-7.

35. Clarke T, Baker P, Watts CJ. Self-harm in adults: a randomised controlled trial of nurse-led management versus routine care only. Journal of Mental Health 2002; 11:167-176.

36. Aoun S. Deliberate self-harm in rural Western Australia: results of an intervention study. Aust N Z J Ment Health Nurs 1999; 8:65-73.

37. Motto JA, Bostrom AG. A randomized controlled trial of postcrisis suicide prevention. Psychiatr Serv 2001; 52:828-33.

38. Morgan HG, Jones EM, Owen JH. Secondary prevention of non-fatal deliberate self-harm. The green card study. Br J Psychiatry 1993; 163:111-2.

39. Evans MO, Morgan HG, Hayward A, Gunnell DJ. Crisis telephone consultation for deliberate self-harm patients: effects on repetition. Br J Psychiatry 1999; 175:23-7.

40. Carter GL, Clover K, Whyte IM, Dawson AH, D'Este C. Postcards from the EDge project: randomised controlled trial of an intervention using postcards to reduce repetition of hospital treated deliberate self poisoning. BMJ 2005; 331:805

41. Walk D. Suicide and community care. Br J Psychiatry 1967; 113:1381-91.

42. Bagley C. The evaluation of a suicide prevention scheme by an ecological method. Soc Sci Med 1968; 2:1-14.

43. Barraclough B, Jennings C, Moss JR. Suicide prevention by the Samaritans. Lancet 1977; 24:868-870.

44. Waterhouse J, Platt S. General hospital admission in the management of parasuicide. A randomised controlled trial. Br J Psychiatry 1990; 156:236-42.

45. Unutzer J, Tang L, Oishi S, Katon W, Williams JWJr, Hunkeler E, et al. Reducing suicidal ideation in depressed older primary care patients. J Am Geriatr Soc 2006; 54:(10)1550-6. Department of Psychiatry, School of Medicine, University of Washington, Seattle, Washington 98195, USA. unutzer@u.washington.edu.

46. Mishara BL, Houle J, Lavoie B. Comparison of the effects of four suicide prevention programs for family and friends of high-risk suicidal men who do not seek help themselves. Suicide Life Threat Behav 2005; 35:(3)329-42. Centre for Research and Intervention on Suicide and Euthanasia, Montreal, Canada. mishara.brian@uqam.ca.

47. Loftin C, McDowall D, Wiersema B, Cottey TJ. Effects of restrictive licensing of handguns on homicide and suicide in the District of Columbia. N Engl J Med 1991; 325:1615-20.

48. Ludwig J, Cook PJ. Homicide and suicide rates associated with implementation of the Brady Handgun Violence Prevention Act. JAMA 2000; 284:585-91.

49. Lott JRJr, Whitley JE. Safe storage gun laws: accidental deaths, suicides, and crime. J Law Econ 2001; 44:6596-6689.

50. Rosengart M, Cummings P, Nathens A, Heagerty P, Maier R, Rivara F. An evaluation of state firearm regulations and homicide and suicide death rates. Inj Prev 2005; 11:77-83.

51. Webster DW, Vernick JS, Zeoli AM, Manganello JA. Association between youth-focused firearm laws and youth suicides. JAMA 2004; 292:594-601.

52. Rich CL, Young JG, Fowler RC, Wagner J, Black NA. Guns and suicide: possible effects of some specific legislation. Am J Psychiatry 1990; 147:342-6.

53. Carrington PJ, Moyer S. Gun control and suicide in Ontario. Am J Psychiatry 1994; 151:606-8.

54. Lester D, Leenaars A. Suicide rates in Canada before and after tightening firearm control laws. Psychol Rep 1993; 72:787-90.

55. Lester D, Leenaars A. Gun control and rates of firearm violence in Canada and the United States: a comment . Canadian Journal of Criminology 1994; 36:463-464.

56. Leenaars AA, Lester D. Gender and the impact of gun control on suicide and homicide. Archives of Suicide Research 1996; 2:223-34.

57. Lester D. Gun availability and the use of guns for suicide and homicide in Canada. Can J Public Health 2000; 91:186-7.

58. Leenaars A, Lester D. The impact of gun control on suicide and homicide across the life span. Canadian Journal of Behavioral Science 1997; 29:1-6.

59. Leenaars AA, Moksony F, Lester D, Wenckstern S. The impact of gun control (Bill C-51) on suicide in Canada. Death Stud 2003; 27:103-24.

60. Bridges FS. Gun control law (Bill C-17), suicide, and homicide in Canada. Psychol Rep 2004; 94:819-26.

61. Cheung AH, Dewa CS. Current trends in youth suicide and firearms regulations. Can J Public Health 2005; 96:131-5.

62. Snowdon J, Harris L. Firearms suicides in Australia. Med J Aust 1992; 156:79-83.

63. Chapman S, Alpers P, Agho K, Jones M. Australia's 1996 gun law reforms: faster falls in firearm deaths, firearm suicides, and a decade without mass shootings. Inj Prev 2006; 12:(6)365-72. School of Public Health, University of Sydney, Sydney, New South Wales, Australia. sc@med.usyd.edu.au.

64. Cantor CH, Slater PJ. The impact of firearm control legislation on suicide in Queensland: preliminary findings. Med J Aust 1995; 162:583-5.

65. Ozanne-Smith J, Ashby K, Newstead S, Stathakis VZ, Clapperton A. Firearm related deaths: the impact of regulatory reform. Inj Prev 2004; 10:280-6.

66. Beautrais AL , Fergusson DM, Horwood LJ. Firearms legislation and reductions in firearm-related suicide deaths in New Zealand. Aust N Z J Psychiatry 2006; 40:(3)253-9. Canterbury Suicide Project, Christchurch School of Medicine & Health Sciences, New Zealand. suicide@chmeds.ac.nz.

67. Prince MI, Thomas SH, James OF, Hudson M. Reduction in incidence of severe paracetamol poisoning. Lancet 2000; 355:2047-8.

68. Turvill JL, Burroughs AK, Moore KP. Change in occurrence of paracetamol overdose in UK after introduction of blister packs. Lancet 2000; 355:2048-9.

69. Robinson D, Smith AM, Johnston GD. Severity of overdose after restriction of paracetamol availability: retrospective study. BMJ 2000; 321:926-7.

70. Sheen CL, Dillon JF, Bateman DN, Simpson KJ, MacDonald TM. Paracetamol-related deaths in Scotland, 1994-2000. Br J Clin Pharmacol 2002; 54:430-2.

71. Hughes B, Durran A, Langford NJ, Mutimer D. Paracetamol poisoning--impact of pack size restrictions. J Clin Pharm Ther 2003; 28:307-10.

72. Hawton K, Townsend E, Deeks J, Appleby L, Gunnell D, Bennewith O, et al. Effects of legislation restricting pack sizes of paracetamol and salicylate on self poisoning in the United Kingdom: before and after study. BMJ 2001; 322:1203-7.

73.   Hawton K. United Kingdom legislation on pack sizes of analgesics: background, ratio-
      nale, and effects on suicide and deliberate self-harm. Suicide Life Threat Behav 2002;
      32:223-9.

74.   Hawton K, Simkin S, Deeks J, Cooper J, Johnston A, Waters K, et al. UK legislation
      on analgesic packs: before and after study of long term effect on poisonings. BMJ 2004;
      329:1076

75.   Morgan O, Griffiths C, Majeed A. Impact of paracetamol pack size restrictions on poi-
      soning from paracetamol in England and Wales: an observational study. J Public Health
      (Oxf) 2005; 27:19-24.

76.   Morgan OW, Griffiths C, Majeed A. Interrupted time-series analysis of regulations to
      reduce paracetamol (acetaminophen) poisoning. PLoS Med 2007; 4:(4)e105 Department
      of Primary Care and Social Medicine, Imperial College London, United Kingdom. omor-
      gan@bigfoot.com.

77.   Donohoe E, Tracey J. Restrictions on sale of paracetamol in Ireland had no impact on the
      number of tablets ingested in acute deliberate overdose. J Toxicol Clin Toxicol 2001; 38
      :251

78.   Balit CR, Isbister GK, Peat J, Dawson AH, Whyte IM. Paracetamol recall: a natural ex-
      periment influencing analgesic poisoning. Med J Aust 2002; 176:162-5.

79.   Kreitman N. The coal gas story. United Kingdom suicide rates, 1960-71. Br J Prev Soc
      Med 1976; 30:86-93.

80.   Kendell RE. Catalytic converters and prevention of suicides. Lancet 1998; 352:1525

81.   Amos T, Appleby L, Kiernan K. Changes in rates of suicide by car exhaust asphyxiation
      in England and Wales. Psychol Med 2001; 31:935-9.

82.   Routley VH, Ozanne-Smith J. The impact of catalytic converters on motor vehicle ex-
      haust gas suicides. Med J Aust 1998; 168:65-7.

83.   Oliver RG, Hetzel BS. Rise and fall of suicide rates in Australia: relation to sedative
      availability. Med J Aust 1972; 2:919-23.

84.   Whitlock FA. Suicide in Brisbane, 1956 to 1973: the drug-death epidemic. Med J Aust
      1975; 1:737-43.

85.   Beautrais AL. Effectiveness of barriers at suicide jumping sites: a case study. Aust N Z J
      Psychiatry 2001; 35:557-62.

86.   Motto JA. Newspaper influence on suicide. A controlled study. Arch Gen Psychiatry
      1970; 23:143-8.

87.   Green LW, Glasgow RE. Evaluating the relevance, generalization, and applicability of
      research: issues in external validation and translation methodology. Eval Health Prof
      2006; 29:126-53.

88. Morgan O, Majeed A. Restricting paracetamol in the United Kingdom to reduce poisoning: a systematic review. J Public Health (Oxf) 2005; 27:12-8.

89. Hawton K, Townsend E, Arensman E, Gunnell D, Hazell P, House Aea. Psychosocial and pharmacological treatments for deliberate self harm (Cochrane Review). In: Anonymous The Cochran Library, Issue 3, 2002. Oxford: Update Software, 2002:

90. Crawford MJ, Thomas O, Khan N, Kulinskaya E. Psychosocial interventions following self-harm: systematic review of their efficacy in preventing suicide. Br J Psychiatry 2007; 190:11-7.

91. Lester D. The effectiveness of suicide prevention centers: a review. Suicide Life Threat Behav 1997; 27:304-10.

92. Isacsson G, Rich CL. Antidepressant drug use and suicide prevention. Int Rev Psychiatry 2005; 17:(3)153-62. Department of Clinical Neuroscience, Division of Psychiatry, Karolinska Institute, Karolinska University Hospital, Huddinge M59, S-141 86 Stockholm, Sweden. Goran.Isaacson@cns.ki.se.

93. Baldessarini RJ, Tondo L, Davis P, Pompili M, Goodwin FK, Hennen J. Decreased risk of suicides and attempts during long-term lithium treatment: a meta-analytic review. Bipolar Disord 2006; 8:625-39.

94. Hennen J, Baldessarini RJ. Suicidal risk during treatment with clozapine: a meta-analysis. Schizophr Res 2005; 73:139-45.

95. Aguilar EJ, Siris SG. Do antipsychotic drugs influence suicidal behavior in schizophrenia? Psychopharmacol Bull 2007; 40:128-42.

96. Bryan CJ, Rudd MD. Advances in the assessment of suicide risk. J Clin Psychol 2006; 62:185-200.

APPENDIX A. DATA COLLECTION FORMS

VA ESP – SUICIDE PREVENTION
PRE SCREENER

Article ID:_____

Final 06/25/08

Reviewer:

Date:

Country (check one)

❑ US
❑ UK/New Zealand/Canada/Australia
❑ Other

Population (check all that apply)
❑ Men
❑ Women

❑ Veterans
❑ Military

Interventions (check all that apply)

❑ Physician
❑ Patient
❑ Population Based

Age (complete all that are reported)

Mean: _____

Median: _____

Range: _____

❑ Organizational
❑ Not stated / Not reported / Not applicable

Outcome (check all)

❑ Attempters
❑ Completers
❑ SI

Setting (check all)
❑ Primary Care
❑ Hospital
❑ Psychiatric

❑ Population Based
❑ Other
❑ Not stated / Not reported / Not applicable

Design (check one)

❑ Experimental
❑ Observational

Intervention Codes

References to Retrieve: _____ _____ _____

_____ _____ _____

_____ _____ _____

Study Design: _____

_____ _____ _____

51

Article ID

Reviewer: Steven Bagley **Assigned on:**

1. **Was the study:**

(Check all
that apply)

Outpatient.............................☐
Inpatient ....☐
Emergency Dept/ Crisis Services....☐
Not reported/Not applicable...........☐

2. **What was the sample size:** (NR for not reported)

	F/Up Duration	Units	Enrolled
Time 0			_____
F/Up 1	_____	_____	_____
F/Up 2	_____	_____	_____
F/Up 3	_____	_____	_____
F/Up 4	_____	_____	_____

Units
1. Days
2. Weeks
3. Months
4. Years
5. NR

3. **Eligibility Criteria**

_____

4. **The intervention consisted of:**

_____

Quality Measurement (only interventions)

1. **Was the study described as randomized?**

Yes...........................☐
No............................☐
Don't know..............☐

2. **Treatment Allocation**
   a. **Was a method of randomization performed?**

Yes...........................☐
No............................☐
Don't know..............☐

   b. **Was the treatment allocation concealed?**

Yes...........................☐
No............................☐
Don't know..............☐

3. **Were the groups similar at baseline regarding the most important prognostic indicators?**

Yes...........................☐
No............................☐
Don't know..............☐

4. **Were the eligibility criteria specified?**

Yes...........................☐
No............................☐
Don't know.............☐

5. **Was the outcome assessor blinded?**

Yes...........................☐
No............................☐
Don't know.............☐

6. **Was the care provider blinded?**

Yes...........................☐
No............................☐
Don't know.............☐

7. **Were subjects blinded?**

Yes...........................☐
No............................☐
Don't know.............☐

8. **Were point estimates and measures of variability presented for the primary outcome measures?**

Yes...........................☐
No............................☐
Don't know.............☐

9. **Were all randomized participants analyzed in the group to which they were allocated?**

Yes...........................☐
No............................☐
Don't know.............☐

10. **Were co-interventions avoided or similar?**

Yes...........................☐
No............................☐
Don't know.............☐

11. **Was the compliance acceptable in all groups?**

Yes...........................☐
No............................☐
Don't know.............☐

12. **Was the drop-out rate described and acceptable?**

Yes...........................☐
No............................☐
Don't know.............☐

13. **Was the timing of the outcome assessment in all groups similar?**

Yes...........................☐
No............................☐
Don't know.............☐

APPENDIX B. EXCLUDED STUDIES

EXCLUDED AFTER INITIAL REVIEW

No Intervention

Cooper, S. L. ; Lezotte, D.; Jacobellis, J., and Diguiseppi, C. Does availability of mental health resources prevent recurrent suicidal behavior? An ecological analysis. Suicide Life Threat Behav. 2006; 36(4):409-17.

Ettlinger, RW. Suicides in a groupd of patients who had previously attempted suicide. Acta Psychiatr Scand. 1964; 40:363-78.

Greer, S. and Lee, H. A. Subsequent progress of potentially lethal attempted suicides. Acta Psychiatr Scand. 1967; 43(4):361-71.

Kessel, N. and McCulloch, W. Repeated acts of self-poisoning and self-injury. Proc R Soc Med. 1966 Feb; 59(2):89-92.

Shah, A. and Bhat, R. Are elderly suicide rates improved by increased provision of mental health service resources? A cross-national study. Int Psychogeriatr. 2008; 1-8.

Foreign Language

Nielsen, A. S. and Nielsen, B. Pattern of choice in preparation of attempted suicide by poisoning--with particular reference to changes in the pattern of prescriptions. Ugeskr Laeger. 1992 Jul 6; 154(28):1972-6.

Rueegsegger, P. Attempted suicide. Clinical statistically and catamnestic studies of 132 attempted suicide patients in Basle University Psychiatric Clinic. 1963;146:81-104.

Duplicate Data

Bateman, A. and Fonagy, P. Treatment of borderline personality disorder with psychoanalytically oriented partial hospitalization: an 18-month follow-up. Am J Psychiatry. 2001 Jan; 158(1):36-42.

McMain, S. Dialectic behaviour therapy reduces suicide attempts compared with non-behavioural psychotherapy in women with borderline personality disorder. Evid Based Ment Health . 2007; 10(1):18.

World Health Organization (WHO). For which strategies of suicide prevention is there evidence of effectiveness? World Health Organitzation: Health Evidence Network; 2004.

Review or Meta-analysis

Althaus, D. and Hegerl, U. The evaluation of suicide prevention activities: state of the art. World J Biol Psychiatry. 2003 Oct; 4(4):156-65.

Anderson, M. and Jenkins, R. The challenge of suicide prevention - an overview of national strategies. Disease Management & Health Outcomes. 2005; 13245-53.

Baldessarini, R. J.; Tondo, L.; Davis, P.; Pompili, M.; Goodwin, F. K., and Hennen, J. Decreased risk of suicides and attempts during long-term lithium treatment: a meta-analytic review. Bipolar Disord. 2006; 8(5 Pt 2):625-39.

Baldessarini, R. J.; Tondo, L.; Strombom, I. M.; Dominguez, S.; Fawcett, J.; Licinio, J.; Oquendo, M. A.; Tollefson, G. D.; Valuck, R. J., and Tohen, M. Ecological studies of antidepressant treatment and suicidal risks. Harv Rev Psychiatry. 2007; 15(4):133-45.

Beautrais, A. ; Fergusson, D.; Coggan, C.; Collings, C.; Doughty, C.; Ellis, P.; Hatcher, S.; Horwood, J.; Merry, S.; Mulder, R.; Poulton, R., and Surgenor, L. Effective strategies for suicide prevention in New Zealand: a review of the evidence. N Z Med J. 2007; 120(1251):U2459 .

Boscarino, J. A. External-cause mortality after psychologic trauma: the effects of stress exposure and predisposition. Compr Psychiatry. 2006; 47(6):503-14.

Chan, J.; Draper, B., and Banerjee, S. Deliberate self-harm in older adults: a review of the literature from 1995 to 2004. Int J Geriatr Psychiatry. 2007; 22(8):720-32.

Cipriani, A.; Pretty, H.; Hawton, K., and Geddes, J. R. Lithium in the prevention of suicidal behavior and all-cause mortality in patients with mood disorders: a systematic review of randomized trials. Am J Psychiatry. 2005; 162(10):1805-19.

Conwell, Y. and Thompson, C. Suicidal behavior in elders. Psychiatr Clin North Am. 2008; 31(2):333-56.

Crawford, M. J.; Thomas, O.; Khan, N., and Kulinskaya, E. Psychosocial interventions following self-harm: systematic review of their efficacy in preventing suicide. Br J Psychiatry. 2007 Jan; 190:11-7.

Daigle, M. S. Suicide prevention through means restriction: assessing the risk of substitution. A critical review and synthesis. Accid Anal Prev. 2005; 37(4):625-32.

Dew, M. A.; Bromet, E. J.; Brent, D., and Greenhouse, J. B. A quantitative literature review of the effectiveness of suicide prevention centers. J Consult Clin Psychol. 1987 Apr; 55(2):239-44.

Diekstra R.F.W. The prevention of suicidal behaviour: evidence for the efficacy of clinical and community based programs. Int J Ment Health. 1992; 21(3):69-87.

Gaynes, B. N.; West, S. L.; Ford, C. A.; Frame, P.; Klein, J., and Lohr, K. N. Screening for suicide risk in adults: a summary of the evidence for the U.S. Preventive Services Task Force. Ann Intern Med. 2004 May 18; 140(10):822-35.

Goldney, R. D. Suicide prevention is possible: a review of recent studies. Archives of Suicide Research. 1998; 4:329-339.

Gunnel, D. and Frankel, S. Prevention of suicide: aspirations and evidence. BMJ. 1994; 308:1227-1233.

Guo, B.; Scott, A., and Bowkers, S. Suicide Prevention Strategies: Evidence from Systematic Reviews. Alberta Heritage Foundation for Medical Research Health Technology Assessment.

Guzzetta, F. ; Tondo, L.; Centorrino, F., and Baldessarini, R. J. Lithium treatment reduces suicide risk in recurrent major depressive disorder. J Clin Psychiatry. 2007; 68(3):380-3.

Hawkins, L. C.; Edwards, J. N., and Dargan, P. I. Impact of restricting paracetamol pack sizes on paracetamol poisoning in the United Kingdom: a review of the literature. Drug Saf. 2007; 30(6):465-79.

Hawton, K.; Townsend, E.; Arensman, E.; Gunnell, D.; Hazell, P., and House, A. et al. Psychosocial and pharmacological treatments for deliberate self harm (Cochrane Review). The Cochran Library, Issue 3, 2002. Oxford: Update Software; 2002.

Heisel, M. J. Suicide and its prevention among older adults. Can J Psychiatry. 2006; 51(3):143-54.

Hirsch, J. K. A review of the literature on rural suicide: risk and protective factors, incidence, and prevention. Crisis. 2006; 27(4):189-99.

Hirsch, S. R.; Walsh, C., and Draper, R. Parasuicide. A review of treatment interventions. J Affect Disord. 1982 Dec; 4(4):299-311.

Isacsson, G. and Rich, C. L. Antidepressant drug use and suicide prevention. Int Rev Psychiatry. 2005; 17(3):153-62.

Lester, D. The effectiveness of suicide prevention centers: a review. Suicide Life Threat Behav. 1997 Fall; 27(3):304-10.

Links, P. S. and Hoffman, B. Preventing suicidal behaviour in a general hospital psychiatric service: priorities for programming. Can J Psychiatry. 2005; 50(8):490-6.

Mackenzie, M.; Blamey, A.; Halliday, E.; Maxwell, M.; McCollam, A.; McDaid, D.; MacLean, J.; Woodhouse, A., and Platt, S. Measuring the tail of the dog that doesn't bark in the night: the case of the national evaluation of Choose Life (the national strategy and action plan to prevent suicide in Scotland). BMC Public Health. 2007; 7146.

Mann, J. J.; Apter, A.; Bertolote, J.; Beautrais, A.; Currier, D.; Haas, A.; Hegerl, U.; Lonnqvist, J.; Malone, K.; Marusic, A.; Mehlum, L.; Patton, G.; Phillips, M.; Rutz, W.; Rihmer, Z.; Schmidtke, A.; Shaffer, D.; Silverman, M.; Takahashi, Y.; Varnik, A.; Wasserman, D.; Yip, P., and Hendin, H. Suicide prevention strategies: a systematic review. JAMA. 2005 Oct 26; 294(16):2064-74.

Moller, H. J. Evidence for beneficial effects of antidepressants on suicidality in depressive patients: a systematic review. Eur Arch Psychiatry Clin Neurosci. 2006; 256(6):329-43.

Morgan, O. and Majeed, A. Restricting paracetamol in the United Kingdom to reduce poisoning: a systematic review. J Public Health (Oxf). 2005 Mar; 27(1):12-8.

NHS Centre for Reviews and Dissemination. Deliberate self-harm. Effective Health Care. 1998; 4(6):1-12.

Pignone, M. P.; Gaynes, B. N.; Rushton, J. L.; Burchell, C. M.; Orleans, C. T.; Mulrow, C. D., and Lohr, K. N. Screening for depression in adults: a summary of the evidence for the U.S. Preventive Services Task Force. Ann Intern Med. 2002 May 21; 136(10):765-76.

Pinkis, J.; Blood, W., and Beautrais, A. et al. Media guidelines on the reporting of suicide. Crisis . 2006; 27(2):82-7.

Rehkopf, D. H. and Buka, S. L. The association between suicide and the socio-economic characteristics of geographical areas: a systematic review. Psychol Med. 2006; 36(2):145-57.

Ritchie, E. C.; Keppler, W. C., and Rothberg, J. M. Suicidal admissions in the United States military. Mil Med. 2003 Mar; 168(3):177-81.

Rodgers, P. L.; Sudak, H. S.; Silverman, M. M., and Litts, D. A. Evidence-based practices project for suicide prevention. Suicide Life Threat Behav. 2007 Apr; 37(2):154-64.

Safer, D. J. and Zito, J. M. Do antidepressants reduce suicide rates? Public Health. 2007; 121(4):274-7.

Seguin, M.; Lesage, A. D.; Turecki, G., and et al. Research project on deaths by suicide in New Brunswick between April 2002 and May 2003. Douglas Hospital Research Centre and New Brunswick Department of Health; 2005.

Staal, M. A. The assessment and prevention of suicide for the 21st century: the Air Force's community awareness training model. Mil Med. 2001 Mar; 166(3):195-8.

Stander, V. A.; Hilton, S. M.; Kennedy, K. R., and Robbins, D. L. Surveillance of completed suicide in the Department of the Navy. Mil Med. 2004 Apr; 169(4):301-6.

van der Sande, R.; Buskens, E.; Allart, E.; van der Graaf, Y., and van Engeland, H. Psychosocial intervention following suicide attempt: a systematic review of treatment interventions. Acta Psychiatr Scand. 1997 Jul; 96(1):43-50.

No Outcome of Interest or Usable Outcome

Preventing patient suicide. Healthc Hazard Manage Monit. 2007; 21(1):1-8.

S-kit Suicide prevention local implementation framework: A strategic multi-agency toolkit aimed at saving lives. National Institute for Mental Health in England, Care Services Improvement Partnership.

Aguilar, E. J. and Siris, S. G. Do antipsychotic drugs influence suicidal behavior in schizophrenia? Psychopharmacol Bull. 2007; 40(3):128-42.

Akroyd, S. and Wyllie, J. Impacts of National Media Campaign to Counter Stigma and Discriminantion Associated with Mental Illness: Survey 4. Wellington, New Zealand: New Zealand Ministry of Health; 2002; Publication 9-20-0004.

Anderson, M. and Jenkins, R. The national suicide prevention strategy for England: the reality of a national strategy for the nursing profession. J Psychiatr Ment Health Nurs. 2006; 13(6):641-50.

Bateman, D. N.; Bain, M.; Gorman, D., and Murphy, D. Changes in paracetamol, antidepressants and opioid poisoning in Scotland during the 1990s. QJM. 2003 Feb; 96(2):125-32.

Beautrais, A. L. Subsequent mortality in medically serious suicide attempts: a 5 year follow-up. Aust N Z J Psychiatry. 2003 Oct; 37(5):595-9.

Bodner, E.; Ben-Artzi, E., and Kaplan, Z. Soldiers who kill themselves: the contribution of dispositional and situational factors. Arch Suicide Res. 2006; 10(1):29-43.

Brent, D. A. and Mann, J. J. Family genetic studies, suicide, and suicidal behavior. Am J Med Genet C Semin Med Genet. 2005 Feb 15; 133(1):13-24.

Bridges, F. S. and Kunselman, J. C. Gun availability and use of guns for suicide, homicide, and murder in Canada. Percept Mot Skills. 2004 Apr; 98(2):594-8.

Burgess, P.; Pirkis, J.; Jolley, D.; Whiteford, H., and Saxena, S. Do nations' mental health policies, programs and legislation influence their suicide rates? An ecological study of 100 countries. Aust N Z J Psychiatry. 2004 Nov-2004 Dec 31; 38(11-12):933-9.

Carrington, P. Gender, gun control, suicide, and homicide in Canada. Archives of Suicide Research. 1999; 5:71-75.

Chan, T. Y. Improvements in the packaging of drugs and chemicals may reduce the likelihood of severe intentional poisonings in adults. Hum Exp Toxicol. 2000 Jul; 19(7):387-91.

Copley, G. B. Epidemiologica risk factors for suicide and attempted suicide in the U.S. Air Force: using administrative data systems and multiple case of death information to improve prevention policy. Diss Abst Int B Sci Eng. 2001; 62807.

Crane, C.; Hawton, K.; Simkin, S., and Coulter, P. Suicide and the media: pitfalls and prevention. Report on a meeting organized by the Reuters Foundation Program at Green College and University of Oxford Centre for Suicide Research at Green College, Oxford, UK, November 18, 2003. Crisis. 2005; 26(1):42-7.

Crome, P. The toxicity of drugs used for suicide. Acta Psychiatr Scand Suppl. 1993; 371:33-7.

Dargan, P. and Jones, A. Effects of legislation restricting pack sizes of paracetamol on self poisoning. It's too early to tell yet. BMJ. 2001 Sep 15; 323(7313):633.

Deutsch, S. and Alt, F. The effect of Massachusetts' gun control law on gun-related crimes in the city of Boston. Evaluation Quarterly. 1977; 1:543-568.

Eaton, K. M. ; Messer, S. C.; Garvey Wilson, A. L., and Hoge, C. W. Strengthening the validity of population-based suicide rate comparisons: an illustration using U.S. military and civilian data. Suicide Life Threat Behav. 2006; 36(2):182-91.

Feightner J and Canadian Task Force on the Periodic Health Examination. Canadian Guide to Clinical Preventitive Health Care. Ottawa, Ontario: Health Canada; 1994.

Florkowski, A.; Gruszczynski, W., and Wawrzyniak, Z. Evaluation of psychopathological factors and origins of suicides committed by soldiers, 1989 to 1998. Mil Med. 2001 Jan; 166(1):44-7.

Gibbons, R. D.; Hur, K.; Bhaumik, D. K., and Mann, J. J. The relationship between antidepressant medication use and rate of suicide. Arch Gen Psychiatry. 2005 Feb; 62(2):165-72.

Gilbody, S.; Whitty, P.; Grimshaw, J., and Thomas, R. Educational and organizational interventions to improve the management of depression in primary care: a systematic review. JAMA. 2003 Jun 18; 289(23):3145-51.

Giles-Sims, J. and Lockhart, C. Explaining cross-state differences in elderly suicide rates and identifying state-level public policy responses that reduce rates. Suicide Life Threat Behav. 2006; 36(6):694-708.

Goldney, R. D.; Fisher, L. J., and Wilson, D. H. Mental health literacy: an impediment to the optimum treatment of major depression in the community. J Affect Disord. 2001 May; 64(2-3):277-84.

Greer, S. and Bagley, C. Effect of psychiatric intervention in attempted suicide: a controlled study. Br Med J. 1971 Feb 6; 1(5744):310-2.

Grossman, D. C.; Mueller, B. A.; Riedy, C.; Dowd, M. D.; Villaveces, A.; Prodzinski, J.; Nakagawara, J.; Howard, J.; Thiersch, N., and Harruff, R. Gun storage practices and risk of youth suicide and unintentional firearm injuries. JAMA. 2005 Feb 9; 293(6):707-14.

Gunnell, D.; Middleton, N., and Frankel, S. Method availability and the prevention of suicide--a re-analysis of secular trends in England and Wales 1950-1975. Soc Psychiatry Psychiatr Epidemiol. 2000 Oct; 35(10):437-43.

Hannaford, P. C.; Thompson, C., and Simpson, M. Evaluation of an educational programme to improve the recognition of psychological illness by general practitioners. Br J Gen Pract. 1996 Jun; 46(407):333-7.

Hartl, T. L. ; Rosen, C.; Drescher, K.; Lee, T. T., and Gusman, F. Predicting high-risk behaviors in veterans with posttraumatic stress disorder. J Nerv Ment Dis. 2005; 193(7):464-72.

Hawton, K.; Simkin, S., and Deeks, J. Co-proxamol and suicide: a study of national mortality statistics and local non-fatal self poisonings. BMJ. 2003 May 10; 326(7397):1006-8.

Hegerl, U.; Althaus, D., and Stefanek, J. Public attitudes towards treatment of depression: effects of an information campaign. Pharmacopsychiatry. 2003 Nov; 36(6):288-91.

Henkel, V.; Mergl, R.; Kohnen, R.; Maier, W.; Moller, H. J., and Hegerl, U. Identifying depression in primary care: a comparison of different methods in a prospective cohort study. BMJ. 2003 Jan 25; 326(7382):200-1.

Hirschfeld, R. M.; Keller, M. B.; Panico, S.; Arons, B. S.; Barlow, D.; Davidoff, F.; Endicott, J.; Froom, J.; Goldstein, M.; Gorman, J. M.; Marek, R. G.; Maurer, T. A.; Meyer, R.; Phillips, K.; Ross, J.; Schwenk, T. L.; Sharfstein, S. S.; Thase, M. E., and Wyatt, R. J. The National Depressive and Manic-Depressive Association consensus statement on the undertreatment of depression. JAMA. 1997 Jan 22-1997 Jan 29; 277(4):333-40.

Isbister, G. and Balit, C. Effects of legislation restricting pack sizes of paracetamol on self poisoning. Authors did not look at effects on all deliberate and accidental self poisoning. BMJ. 2001 Sep 15; 323(7313):633-4.

Jorm, A. F.; Christensen, H., and Griffiths, K. M. The impact of beyondblue: the national depression initiative on the Australian public's recognition of depression and beliefs about treatments. Aust N Z J Psychiatry. 2005 Apr; 39(4):248-54.

Kaleveld, L. and English, B. Evaluating a suicide prevention program: a question of impact. Health Promot J Austr. 2005 Aug; 16(2):129-33.

Kapur, S.; Mieczkowski, T., and Mann, J. J. Antidepressant medications and the relative risk of suicide attempt and suicide. JAMA. 1992 Dec 23-1992 Dec 30; 268(24):3441-5.

Kelly, C. The effects of depression awareness seminars on general practitioners knowledge of depressive illness. Ulster Med J. 1998 May; 67(1):33-5.

Kelly, S. and Bunting, J. Trends in suicide in England and Wales, 1982-96. Popul Trends. 1998 Summer; (92):29-41.

Kennedy, P. Efficacy of a regional poisoning treatment centre in preventing further suicidal behaviour. Br Med J. 1972 Nov 4; 4(5835):255-7.

Laing, W.; Gordon, L.; Lee, D.; Good, A., and Bateman, D. Have the new pack size regulations impacted on UK paracetamol overdose? J Toxicol Clin Toxicol. 2001; 39:301.

Lester, D. Firearm availability and use of firearms for suicide and homicide. Perceptual and Motor Skills. 2000; 91:758.

Lin, E. H.; Simon, G. E.; Katzelnick, D. J., and Pearson, S. D. Does physician education on depression management improve treatment in primary care? J Gen Intern Med. 2001 Sep; 16(9):614-9.

Luoma, J. B.; Martin, C. E., and Pearson, J. L. Contact with mental health and primary care providers before suicide: a review of the evidence. Am J Psychiatry. 2002 Jun; 159(6):909-16.

Mahon, M. J. ; Tobin, J. P.; Cusack, D. A.; Kelleher, C., and Malone, K. M. Suicide among regular-duty military personnel: a retrospective case-control study of occupation-specific risk factors for workplace suicide. Am J Psychiatry. 2005; 162(9):1688-96.

Marzuk, P. M.; Leon, A. C.; Tardiff, K.; Morgan, E. B.; Stajic, M., and Mann, J. J. The effect of access to lethal methods of injury on suicide rates. Arch Gen Psychiatry. 1992 Jun; 49(6):451-8.

McClure, G. M. Changes in suicide in England and Wales, 1960-1997. Br J Psychiatry. 2000 Jan; 176:64-7.

McLeavey, B. C.; Daly, R. J.; Ludgate, J. W., and Murray, C. M. Interpersonal problem-solving skills training in the treatment of self-poisoning patients. Suicide Life Threat Behav. 1994 Winter; 24(4):382-94.

Miller, M.; Hemenway, D., and Azrael, D. Firearms and suicide in the northeast. J Trauma. 2004 Sep; 57(3):626-32.

Mills, P. D. ; Neily, J.; Luan, D.; Osborne, A., and Howard, K. Actions and implementation strategies to reduce suicidal events in the Veterans Health Administration. Jt Comm J Qual Patient Saf. 2006; 32(3):130-41.

Ministry of Health. Suicide and the Media: The Reporting and Portrayal of suicide in the Media. Wellington: Ministry of Health; 1999.

Mundt, R. J. Gun control and rates of firearms violence in Canada and the United States. Canadian Journal of Criminology. 1990; 32:137-154.

Naismith, S. L.; Hickie, I. B.; Scott, E. M., and Davenport, T. A. Effects of mental health training and clinical audit on general practitioners' management of common mental disorders. Med J Aust. 2001 Jul 16; 175 Suppl:S42-7.

Paykel, E. S.; Hart, D., and Priest, R. G. Changes in public attitudes to depression during the Defeat Depression Campaign. Br J Psychiatry. 1998 Dec; 173:519-22.

Pettit, J. W.; Paukert, A. L.; Joiner, T. E. Jr., and Rudd, M. D. Pilot sample of very early onset bipolar disorder in a military population moderates the association of negative life events and non-fatal suicide attempt. Bipolar Disord. 2006; 8(5 Pt 1):475-84.

Pfaff, J. J.; Acres, J. G., and McKelvey, R. S. Training general practitioners to recognise and respond to psychological distress and suicidal ideation in young people. Med J Aust. 2001 Mar 5; 174(5):222-6.

Platt, S.; McLean, J.; McCollam, A.; Blamey, A.; Mackenzie, M.; McDaid, D.; Maxwell, M.; Halliday, E., and Woodhouse, A. Evaluation of the first phase of Choose Life: the National Strategy and Action Plan to Prevent Suicide in Scotland 2006. Edinburgh: Scottish Executive Social Research.

Rabasca, L. Military suicide-prevention program reduces the stigma of seeking help. Am Psychol Assoc Monitor. 1999; 30(9):8.

Rihmer, Z.; Belso, N., and Kalmar, S. Antidepressants and suicide prevention in Hungary. Acta Psychiatr Scand. 2001 Mar; 103(3):238-9.

Sakinofsky, I. The current evidence base for the clinical care of suicidal patients: strengths and weaknesses. Can J Psychiatry. 2007; 52(6 Suppl 1):7S-20S.

Sakinofsky, I. Treating suicidality in depressive illness. Part 2: does treatment cure or cause suicidality? Can J Psychiatry. 2007; 52(6 Suppl 1):85S-101S.

Saunders, K. and Hawton, K. Suicide prevention and audit. Br J Hosp Med (Lond). 2005; 66(11):627-30.

Scarff, E. Evaluation of the Canadian gun control legislation: final report. Ottawa: Canadian Government Publishing Centre; 1983.

Scoville, S. L.; Gubata, M. E.; Potter, R. N.; White, M. J., and Pearse, L. A. Deaths attributed to suicide among enlisted U.S. Armed Forces recruits, 1980-2004. Mil Med. 2007; 172(10):1024-31.

Sheen, C. and Dillon, J. The effect on toxicity and healthcare costs on reducing the size of available acetaminophen pack sizes in the Tayside region of Scotland. Gastroenterology. 2001; 120(Suppl. 1):A-228.

Sheen, C. L.; Dillon, J. F.; Bateman, D. N.; Simpson, K., and MacDonald, T. M. The effect on toxicity on reducing the size of available paracetamol pack sizes. Gut. 2001; 48((Suppl 1)):A105.

Sheen, C. L.; Dillon, J. F.; Bateman, D. N.; Simpson, K. J., and MacDonald, T. M. Paracetamol pack size restriction: the impact on paracetamol poisoning and the over-the-counter supply of paracetamol, aspirin and ibuprofen. Pharmacoepidemiol Drug Saf. 2002 Jun; 11(4):329-31.

Shenassa, E. D.; Rogers, M. L.; Spalding, K. L., and Roberts, M. B. Safer storage of firearms at home and risk of suicide: a study of protective factors in a nationally representative sample. J Epidemiol Community Health. 2004 Oct; 58(10):841-8.

Sloan, J. H.; Rivara, F. P.; Reay, D. T.; Ferris, J. A., and Kellermann, A. L. Firearm regulations and rates of suicide. A comparison of two metropolitan areas. N Engl J Med. 1990 Feb 8; 322(6):369-73.

Sorenson, S. B. and Vittes, K. A. Mental health and firearms in community-based surveys: implications for suicide prevention. Eval Rev. 2008; 32(3):239-56.

Stuart, H. Fighting stigma and discrimination is fighting for mental health. Canadian Public Policy. 2005; S21-S28.

Thoresen, S. and Mehlum, L. Suicide in peacekeepers: risk factors for suicide versus accidental death. Suicide Life Threat Behav. 2006; 36(4):432-42.

Thoresen, S. ; Mehlum, L.; Roysamb, E., and Tonnessen, A. Risk factors for completed suicide in veterans of peacekeeping: repatriation, negative life events, and marital status. Arch Suicide Res. 2006; 10(4):353-63.

Tiet, Q. Q.; Finney, J. W., and Moos, R. H. Recent sexual abuse, physical abuse, and suicide attempts among male veterans seeking psychiatric treatment. Psychiatr Serv. 2006; 57(1):107-13.

Tiet, Q. Q.; Ilgen, M. A.; Byrnes, H. F., and Moos, R. H. Suicide attempts among substance use disorder patients: an initial step toward a decision tree for suicide management. Alcohol Clin Exp Res. 2006; 30(6):998-1005.

Troister, T. ; Links, P. S., and Cutcliffe, J. Review of predictors of suicide within 1 year of discharge from a psychiatric hospital. Curr Psychiatry Rep. 2008; 10(1):60-5.

Unutzer, J.; Katon, W.; Callahan, C. M.; Williams, J. W. Jr; Hunkeler, E.; Harpole, L.; Hoffing, M.; Della Penna, R. D.; Noel, P. H.; Lin, E. H.; Arean, P. A.; Hegel, M. T.; Tang, L.; Belin, T. R.; Oishi, S., and Langston, C. Collaborative care management of late-life depression in the primary care setting: a randomized controlled trial. JAMA. 2002 Dec 11; 288(22):2836-45.

Valentini, W.; Levav, I.; Kohn, R.; Miranda, C. T.; Mello, A. A.; Mello, M. F., and Ramos, C. P. [An educational training program for physicians for diagnosis and treatment of depression]. Rev Saude Publica. 2004 Aug; 38(4):522-8.

Voaklander, D. C.; Rowe, B. H.; Dryden, D. M.; Pahal, J.; Saar, P., and Kelly, K. D. Medical illness, medication use and suicide in seniors: a population-based case-control study. Epidemiol Community Health. 2008; 62(2):138-46.

Vuorilehto, M. S.; Melartin, T. K., and Isometsa, E. T. Suicidal behaviour among primary-care patients with depressive disorders. Psychol Med. 2006; 36(2):203-10.

Zivin, K.; Kim, H. M.; McCarthy, J. F.; Austin, K. L.; Hoggatt, K. J.; Walters, H., and Valenstein, M. Suicide mortality among individuals receiving treatment for depression in the Veterans Affairs health system: associations with patient and treatment setting characteristics. Am J Public Health. 2007; 97(12):2193-8.

Adolescent

Rotheram-Borus, M. J.; Piacentini, J.; Cantwell, C.; Belin, T. R., and Song, J. The 18-month impact of an emergency room intervention for adolescent female suicide attempters. J Consult Clin Psychol. 2000 Dec; 68(6):1081-93.

Design- Other

Appleby, L. and Sherratt, J. Good clinical practice on suicide and suicide prevention. Psychiatr Bull R Coll Psychiatr. 2001; 2541-42.

EXCLUDED AT FURTHER REVIEW (N=49)

Country

Apter, A.; King, R. A.; Bleich, A.; Fluck, A.; Kotler, M., and Kron, S. Fatal and non-fatal suicidal behavior in Israeli adolescent males. Arch Suicide Res. 2008; 12(1):20-9.

Bellanger, M. M.; Jourdain, A., and Batt-Moillo, A. Might the decrease in the suicide rates in France be due to regional prevention programmes? Soc Sci Med. 2007; 65(3):431-41.

Bradvik, L. and Berglund, M. Long-term treatment and suicidal behavior in severe depression: ECT and antidepressant pharmacotherapy may have different effects on the occurrence and seriousness of suicide attempts. Depress Anxiety. 2006; 23(1):34-41.

Cedereke, M.; Monti, K., and Ojehagen, A. Telephone contact with patients in the year after a suicide attempt: does it affect treatment attendance and outcome? A randomised controlled study. Eur Psychiatry. 2002 Apr; 17(2):82-91.

De Leo, D.; Dello Buono, M., and Dwyer, J. Suicide among the elderly: the long-term impact of a telephone support and assessment intervention in northern Italy. Br J Psychiatry. 2002 Sep; 181:226-9.

Dieserud, G.; Loeb, M., and Ekeberg, O. Suicidal behavior in the municipality of Baerum, Norway: a 12-year prospective study of parasuicide and suicide. Suicide Life Threat Behav. 2000 Spring; 30(1):61-73.

Gunnell, D.; Fernando, R.; Hewagama, M.; Priyangika, W. D.; Konradsen, F., and Eddleston, M. The impact of pesticide regulations on suicide in Sri Lanka. Int J Epidemiol. 2007.

Hegerl, U.; Althaus, D.; Schmidtke, A., and Niklewski, G. The alliance against depression: 2-year evaluation of a community-based intervention to reduce suicidality. Psychol Med. 2006 Sep; 36(9):1225-33.

Kapusta, N. D.; Etzersdorfer, E.; Krall, C., and Sonneck, G. Firearm legislation reform in the European Union: impact on firearm availability, firearm suicide and homicide rates in Austria. Br J Psychiatry. 2007; 191 253-7.

Matakas, F. and Rohrbach, E. Suicide prevention in the psychiatric hospital. Suicide Life Threat Behav. 2007; 37(5):507-17.

Ohberg, A.; Lonnqvist, J.; Sarna, S.; Vuori, E., and Penttila, A. Trends and availability of suicide methods in Finland. Proposals for restrictive measures. Br J Psychiatry. 1995 Jan; 166(1):35-43.

Oyama, H.; Fujita, M.; Goto, M.; Shibuya, H., and Sakashita, T. Outcomes of community-based screening for depression and suicide prevention among Japanese elders. Gerontologist. 2006 Dec; 46(6):821-6.

Oyama, H.; Goto, M.; Fujita, M.; Shibuya, H., and Sakashita, T. Preventing elderly suicide through primary care by community-based screening for depression in rural Japan. Crisis. 2006; 27(2):58-65.

Oyama, H.; Koida, J.; Sakashita, T., and Kudo, K. Community-based prevention for suicide in elderly by depression screening and follow-up. Community Ment Health J. 2004 Jun; 40(3):249-63.

Oyama, H.; Ono, Y.; Watanabe, N.; Tanaka, E.; Kudoh, S.; Sakashita, T.; Sakamoto, S.; Neichi, K.; Satoh, K.; Nakamura, K., and Yoshimura, K. Local community intervention through depression screening and group activity for elderly suicide prevention. Psychiatry Clin Neurosci. 2006; 60(1):110-4.

Oyama, H.; Watanabe, N.; Ono, Y.; Sakashita, T.; Takenoshita, Y.; Taguchi, M.; Takizawa, T.; Miura, R., and Kumagai, K. Community-based suicide prevention through group activity for the elderly successfully reduced the high suicide rate for females. Psychiatry Clin Neurosci. 2005; 59(3):337-44.

Raj, M. A. J.; Kumaraiah, V., and Bhide, A. V. Cognitive-behavioural intervention in deliberate self-harm. Acta Psychiatr Scand. 2001; 104:340-5.

Rutz, W.; von Knorring, L., and Walinder, J. Frequency of suicide on Gotland after systematic postgraduate education of general practitioners. Acta Psychiatr Scand. 1989 Aug; 80(2):151-4.

Szanto, K.; Kalmar, S.; Hendin, H.; Rihmer, Z., and Mann, J. J. A suicide prevention program in a region with a very high suicide rate. Arch Gen Psychiatry. 2007; 64(8):914-20.

Torhorst, A.; Moller, H. J.; Burk, F.; Kurz, A.; Wachtler, C., and Lauter, H. The psychiatric management of parasuicide patients: a controlled clinical study comparing different strategies of outpatient treatment. Crisis. 1987 Mar; 8(1):53-61.

Torhorst, A.; Moller, H. J., and Schimid-Bode, K. W. Comparing a 3-month and a 12-month outpatient aftercare program for parasuicide repeaters. Current Issues of SuicidologyBerlin, Germany: Springer-Verlag; 1988; pp. 19-24.

Vaiva, G.; Vaiva, G.; Ducrocq, F.; Meyer, P.; Mathieu, D.; Philippe, A.; Libersa, C., and Goudemand, M. Effect of telephone contact on further suicide attempts in patients discharged from an emergency department: randomised controlled study. Bmj. 2006; 332(7552):1241-5.

van den Bosch, L. M.; Koeter, M. W.; Stijnen, T. ; Verheul, R., and van den Brink, W. Sustained efficacy of dialectical behaviour therapy for borderline personality disorder. Behav Res Ther. 2005; 43(9):1231-41.

van der Sande, R.; van Rooijen, L.; Buskens, E.; Allart, E.; Hawton, K.; van der Graaf, Y., and van Engeland, H. Intensive in-patient and community intervention versus routine care after attempted suicide. A randomised controlled intervention study. Br J Psychiatry. 1997 Jul; 171:35-41.

Van Heeringen, C.; Jannes, S.; Buylaert, W.; Henderick, H.; De Bacquer, D., and Van Remoor-tel, J. The management of non-compliance with referral to out-patient after-care among attempted suicide patients: a controlled intervention study. Psychol Med. 1995 Sep; 25(5):963-70.

Varnik, A.; Kolves, K.; Vali, M.; Tooding, L. M., and Wasserman, D. Do alcohol restrictions reduce suicide mortality? Addiction. 2007; 102(2):251-6.

Verkes, R. J.; Van der Mast, R. C.; Hengeveld, M. W.; Tuyl, J. P.; Zwinderman, A. H., and Van Kempen, G. M. Reduction by paroxetine of suicidal behavior in patients with repeated suicide attempts but not major depression. Am J Psychiatry. 1998 Apr; 155(4):543-7.

Zonda, T. and Lester, D. Preventing suicide by educating general practitioners. Omega (West-port). 2006; 54(1):53-7.

Pharmacotherapy

Battaglia, J.; Wolff, T. K.; Wagner-Johnson, D. S.; Rush, A. J.; Carmody, T. J., and Basco, M. R. Structured diagnostic assessment and depot fluphenazine treatment of multiple suicide at-tempters in the emergency department. Int Clin Psychopharmacol. 1999 Nov; 14(6):361-72.

Coryell, W.; Arndt, S.; Turvey, C.; Endicott, J.; Solomon, D.; Mueller, T.; Leon, A. C., and Keller, M. Lithium and suicidal behavior in major affective disorder: a case-control study. Acta Psychiatr Scand. 2001 Sep; 104(3):193-7.

Ludwig, J.; Marcotte, D. E., and Norberg, K. Anti-Depressants and Suicide. 2007 Feb.

Montgomery, D. B.; Roberts, A.; Green, M.; Bullock, T.; Baldwin, D., and Montgomery, S. A. Lack of efficacy of fluoxetine in recurrent brief depression and suicidal attempts. Eur Arch Psychiatry Clin Neurosci. 1994; 244(4):211-5.

Montgomery, S.; Cronholm, B.; Asberg, M., and Montgomery, D. B. Differential effects on sui-cidal ideation of mianserin, maprotiline and amitriptyline. Br J Clin Pharmacol. 1978; 5 Suppl 1:77S-80S.

Montgomery, S. A.; Roy, D., and Montgomery, D. B. The prevention of recurrent suicidal acts. Br J Clin Pharmacol. 1983; 15 Suppl 2:183S-188S.

Verkes, R. J.; Van der Mast, R. C.; Hengeveld, M. W.; Tuyl, J. P.; Zwinderman, A. H., and Van Kempen, G. M. Reduction by paroxetine of suicidal behavior in patients with repeated suicide attempts but not major depression. Am J Psychiatry. 1998 Apr; 155(4):543-7.

Psychotherapy

Bateman, A. and Fonagy, P. Effectiveness of partial hospitalization in the treatment of border-line personality disorder: a randomized controlled trial. Am J Psychiatry. 1999 Oct; 156(10):1563-9.

Blum, N.; St John, D.; Pfohl, B.; Stuart, S.; McCormick, B.; Allen, J.; Arndt, S., and Black, D. W. Systems Training for Emotional Predictability and Problem Solving (STEPPS) for outpatients with borderline personality disorder: a randomized controlled trial and 1-year follow-up. Am J Psychiatry. 2008; 165(4):468-78.

Bradvik, L. and Berglund, M. Long-term treatment and suicidal behavior in severe depression: ECT and antidepressant pharmacotherapy may have different effects on the occurrence and seriousness of suicide attempts. Depress Anxiety. 2006; 23(1):34-41.

Evans, K.; Tyrer, P.; Catalan, J.; Schmidt, U.; Davidson, K.; Dent, J.; Tata, P.; Thornton, S.; Barber, J., and Thompson, S. Manual-assisted cognitive-behaviour therapy (MACT): a randomized controlled trial of a brief intervention with bibliotherapy in the treatment of recurrent deliberate self-harm. Psychol Med. 1999 Jan; 29(1):19-25.

Liberman, R. P. and Eckman, T. Behavior therapy vs insight-oriented therapy for repeated suicide attempters. Arch Gen Psychiatry. 1981 Oct; 38(10):1126-30.

Linehan, M. M.; Armstrong, H. E.; Suarez, A.; Allmon, D., and Heard, H. L. Cognitive-behavioral treatment of chronically parasuicidal borderline patients. Arch Gen Psychiatry. 1991 Dec; 48(12):1060-4.

Linehan, M. M.; Comtois, K. A.; Murray, A. M.; Brown, M. Z.; Gallop, R. J.; Heard, H. L.; Korslund, K. E.; Tutek, D. A.; Reynolds, S. K., and Lindenboim, N. Two-year randomized controlled trial and follow-up of dialectical behavior therapy vs therapy by experts for suicidal behaviors and borderline personality disorder. Arch Gen Psychiatry. 2006; 63(7):757-66.

Matakas, F. and Rohrbach, E. Suicide prevention in the psychiatric hospital. Suicide Life Threat Behav. 2007; 37(5):507-17.

Patsiokas, A. T. and Clum, G. A. Effects of psychotherapeutic strategies in the treatment of suicide attempters. Journal of Psychotherapy. 1985; 22(281).

Raj, M. A. J.; Kumaraiah, V., and Bhide, A. V. Cognitive-behavioural intervention in deliberate self-harm. Acta Psychiatr Scand. 2001; 104:340-5.

Rudd, M. D.; Rajab, M. H.; Orman, D. T.; Joiner, T.; Stulman, D. A., and Dixon, W. Effectiveness of an outpatient intervention targeting suicidal young adults: preliminary results. J Consult Clin Psychol. 1996 Feb; 64(1):179-90.

Salkovskis, P. M.; Atha, C., and Storer, D. Cognitive-behavioural problem solving in the treatment of patients who repeatedly attempt suicide. A controlled trial. Br J Psychiatry. 1990 Dec; 157:871-6.

Tarrier, N.; Haddock, G.; Lewis, S.; Drake, R., and Gregg, L. Suicide behaviour over 18 months in recent onset schizophrenic patients: the effects of CBT. Schizophr Res. 2006; 83(1):15-27.

Torhorst, A.; Moller, H. J.; Burk, F.; Kurz, A.; Wachtler, C., and Lauter, H. The psychiatric management of parasuicide patients: a controlled clinical study comparing different strategies of outpatient treatment. Crisis. 1987 Mar; 8(1):53-61.

Tyrer, P.; Thompson, S.; Schmidt, U.; Jones, V.; Knapp, M.; Davidson, K.; Catalan, J.; Airlie, J.; Baxter, S.; Byford, S.; Byrne, G.; Cameron, S.; Caplan, R.; Cooper, S.; Ferguson, B.; Freeman, C.; Frost, S.; Godley, J.; Greenshields, J.; Henderson, J.; Holden, N.; Keech, P.; Kim, L.; Logan, K.; Manley, C.; MacLeod, A.; Murphy, R.; Patience, L.; Ramsay, L.; De Munroz, S.; Scott, J.; Seivewright, H.; Sivakumar, K.; Tata, P.; Thornton, S.; Ukoumunne, O. C., and Wessely, S. Randomized controlled trial of brief cognitive behaviour therapy versus treatment as usual in recurrent deliberate self-harm: the POPMACT study. Psychol Med. 2003 Aug; 33(6):969-76.

van den Bosch, L. M.; Koeter, M. W.; Stijnen, T. ; Verheul, R., and van den Brink, W. Sustained efficacy of dialectical behaviour therapy for borderline personality disorder. Behav Res Ther. 2005; 43(9):1231-41.

Weinberg, I.; Gunderson, J. G.; Hennen, J., and Cutter, C. J. Jr. Manual assisted cognitive treatment for deliberate self-harm in borderline personality disorder patients. J Personal Disord. 2006; 20(5):482-92.

Suicidal Ideation

Bruce, M. L.; Ten Have, T. R.; Reynolds, C. F. 3rd; Katz, I. I.; Schulberg, H. C.; Mulsant, B. H.; Brown, G. K.; McAvay, G. J.; Pearson, J. L., and Alexopoulos, G. S. Reducing suicidal ideation and depressive symptoms in depressed older primary care patients: a randomized controlled trial. JAMA. 2004 Mar 3; 291(9):1081-91.

Montgomery, S.; Cronholm, B.; Asberg, M., and Montgomery, D. B. Differential effects on suicidal ideation of mianserin, maprotiline and amitriptyline. Br J Clin Pharmacol. 1978; 5 Suppl 1:77S-80S.

Patsiokas, A. T. and Clum, G. A. Effects of psychotherapeutic strategies in the treatment of suicide attempters. Journal of Psychotherapy. 1985; 22(281).

Raj, M. A. J.; Kumaraiah, V., and Bhide, A. V. Cognitive-behavioural intervention in deliberate self-harm. Acta Psychiatr Scand. 2001; 104:340-5.

APPENDIX C. EVIDENCE TABLES

Evidence Table 1. Studies Describing Suicide Prevention Interventions in Military Personnel and Veterans

Author, Year	Study Design	Country / Setting	Veteran / Military	Outcome	Intervention	Detailed Intervention	Results
James LC et al 1996[13]	Cohort	US / Population & Other	No / Yes	Completers	Population / Organizational	25th Infantry Division (Light) Suicide Prevention Program implementation beginning in 1992. This program incorporated warning signs and risk factors along with community education.	In the two years following complete implementation (1994) the suicide rate decreased to 3.
McDaniel WW et al. 1990[14]	Cohort	US / Other	No / Yes	Attempters & SI	Organizational	This two year retrospective study examines a suicide prevention program at the training command center aimed at the instructors. The classes, provided in 1986 and then again from June 1987-January 1988, were targeted at informing instructors on how to recognize signs of distress and students at risk.	The average number of suicide attempts was 9.4 per 100,000 per month. The number of instructors who received training was negatively correlated (-0.65, p<0.001) with number of suicide attempts per month.
Knox KL et al. 2003[15]	Interrupted Time Series	US / Population	No / Yes	Completers	Population / Organizational	To assess the impact of the US Air Force suicide prevention program implemented in 1996, this study looked at 5,260,292 air force personnel. The program aimed to reduce risk factors for suicide and enhance protective factors as well as increasing understanding of mental health and policies while decreasing the stigma of seeking mental health assistance.	The relative risk for suicide when comparing the pre-implementation population and post-implementation population was 0.67(95% CI: 0.57, 0.80). There was a 33% relative risk reduction for those in the post implementation group.
Jones DE et al. 2001[16]	Observational	US / Population	No / Yes	Completers	Population	Existing resources (education in suicide awareness and life skills training, counseling, post-suicide interventions, and suicide incident reporting) were augmented with new training video using positive role models to increase detection and referral.	For Navy, suicide rate dropped to 9.2/100000, the lowest rate in 10 years. For the Marine Corps, the rate was 15.6/100000.
Kennedy CH et al. 2005[17]	Cohort	US / Other	No / Yes	Attempters	Patient	This is a one year follow up on a gambling treatment program implemented in January 2003 as a part of the Substance Abuse Rehabilitation Program at the US Naval Hospital in Okinawa, Japan. There was 35 participants.	Prior to treatment 7 participants expressed suicidal ideation and 3 (8.5%) made suicide attempts related to their gambling. Post-implementation, no participants expressed suicidal ideation or attempted suicide.
Rozanov VA et al. 2002[18]	Cohort	Ukraine / Population	No / Yes	Completers	Population / Organizational	This two year suicide prevention program, implemented in 2000, used training seminars for soldiers, professional officers, and commanders that spanned the course of one year. Brochures on suicide prevention were distributed to more than 2000 soldiers.	The average number of suicides per year between 1988 and 1999 was 32.6per 100,000. In 1999 the suicide rate was 74.7per 100,000. During the first year of the program there was no reported suicides and in the 2nd year there were 16.7 per 100,000 reported suicides.
Gordana DJ et al. 2007[19]	Cohort	Serbia & Montenegro / Other	No / Yes	Completers	Organizational	Two year follow up on a Suicide Prevention Program, based on the U.S. Air force suicide prevention program, that was implemented in 2003. The program focused on early prevention and identification of those at increased risk of committing suicide. The long-term objective was modifying military-specific risk factors for suicide. The program was applied by selection, education, and motivation.	Suicides decreased from 15 in 2003 (pre-implementation) to 9 in 2004 and 7 in 2005. After one year of implementation, suicides decreased from 13 per 100,000 of military personnel to 5 per 100,000 military personnel.
Koons CR et al. 2001[22]	RCT	UC / Psychiatric	Yes / No	Attempters & SI	Patient	Dialectical behavior therapy (DBT) in with borderline personality disorder. 28 women veterans were randomized to DBT or usual care groups. 20 patients (10 in each group) completed the treatment.	Patients in the DBT reported significantly greater decrease in depression (as measured by the BDI), suicidal ideation, and hopelessness than usual care patients.
Gibbons RD et al. 2007[24]	Observational	US / Primary Care & Psychiatric	Yes / No	Attempters	Patient	Comparison of 226,866 patients in a VHA data set who were diagnosed with depression and had one of the following treatments: no antidepressant, SSRI, non-SSRI, tricyclic or combinations.	Odds ratio for comparing the SSRI treatment to the no antidepressant, non-SSRI and tricycle categories was 0.34 (95% CI: 0.31 to 0.38, p<0.0001).
Ilgen MA et al. 2007[23]	Observational	US / Psychiatric	Yes / No	Attempters	Patient	This study followed 3733 veterans entering either a residential or outpatient substance abuse program. Data on suicide attempts were collected for 12 months prior to entry, during treatment and 12 months after entry.	During treatment, residential treatment was associated with a lower rate of suicide attempts than outpatient treatment. Predicting suicide attempts after drug abuse treatment was not significant for either setting.

SI: Suicidal Ideation

Evidence Table 2. RCT and CCTs Describing Suicide Interventions

Author, Year	Study Design / Setting	Sample Size Enrolled	Follow Up Time Points / Follow Up	Veterans / Military	Country / Mean Age	Eligibility Criteria	Described as Randomized	Method of Randomization	Allocation Concealment	Similarity at Baseline between groups	Eligibility Criteria Specified	Outcome Assessor Blinded	Care provider blinded	Patients Blinded	Point estimates & measures of variability for primary outcomes variable	Randomized patients analyzed in group they were allocated to	Co-interventions avoided	Compliance acceptable	Drop-out rate described	Timing of Outcome Assessment Similar	Intervention	Duration of Treatment	Outcome	Adverse Events
Koons CJ et al. 2001[22]	RCT / Psychiatric	28	3 mths / NR; 6 mths / 20	Yes / No	US / 35	Female veterans with borderline personality disorder	Yes	Don't Know	Don't Know	Yes	Yes	Yes	No	No	Yes	Yes		Yes	Yes	Yes	dialectical behavior therapy (DBT) and treatment as usual (TAU)	weekly meetings of 90 minutes each?	Attempters & SI	30% in DBT, 20% in TAU at post treatment reported self harm
Welu T 1977[25]	RCT / Psychiatric	120	4 mths / 119	No / No	US / 29	ED contact for suicide attempt	Yes	Yes	Don't Know	Don't Know	Yes	Don't Know	No	No	Yes	Yes	Yes	Don't Know	Yes	Yes	follow up outreach program by therapists	4 month follow up outreach program	Attempters	at 4 months there were 3 repeated attempts in experimental group & 9 in control
Termansen PE et al. 1975[26]	CCT / Psychiatric	202	3 mths / 128	No / No	Canada / NR	ER presentation for suicide attempt	No	No	No	Don't Know	Yes	No	No	No	Yes	Yes	Don't Know	No	Yes	Yes	1. Mental health follow up 2. Phone follow up 3. Reassessment at 3 mths. 4. assessment at 3 mths.	12 weeks	Attempters	Reattempt rate, 1: 2.2%, 2: 6.1%, 3: 22%, 4: 11%
Allard R et al. 1992[27]	RCT / Psychiatric	150	12 mths / NR; 18 mths / NR; 24 mths / 126	No / No	Canada / NR	Seen in ED after suicide attempt	Yes	Don't Know	Don't Know	Yes	Yes	Don't Know	No	No	Yes	Yes	Don't Know	Yes	Yes	Yes	a treatment plan, follow up visits, one home visit, reminder for missed appointments. Treatment could include meds or therapy	18 therapy sessions & a home visit over 1 year	Attempters & Completers	3 suicides in experimental & 1 in control

Evidence Table 2. RCT and CCTs Describing Suicide Interventions Continued

Author, Year	Study Design / Setting	Sample Size Enrolled	Follow Up Time Points / Follow Up	Veterans / Military	Country / Mean Age	Eligibility Criteria	Described as Randomized	Method of Randomization	Allocation Concealment	Similarity at Baseline between groups	Eligibility Criteria Specified	Outcome Assessor Blinded	Care provider blinded	Patients Blinded	Point estimates & measures of variability for primary outcomes variable	Randomized patients analyzed in group they were allocated to	Co-interventions avoided	Compliance acceptable	Drop-out rate described	Timing of Outcome Assessment Similar	Intervention	Duration of Treatment	Outcome	Adverse Events
Chowdhury N et al. 1973[28]	CCT / Psychiatric	155	6 mths / NR	No / No	UK / NR	Hospital contact for deliberate self harm for repeat patients	No	No	Don't Know	Yes	Yes	Don't Know	No	No	Yes		Don't Know	Don't Know		Yes	outpatient clinic, home visits, telephone hotline	6 months from discharge	Attempters	24% acts of parasuicide in treatment & 23% in control 10% repeat
Gardner R et al. 1977[29]	RCT / Hospital	312	1 yr / 273	No / No	UK / NR	Patient admitted to hospital for self poisoning		Don't Know	Yes	Yes / Don't Know	Yes	Yes	Yes	No	Yes	Yes	Don't Know	Yes	Yes	Yes	Inpatient assessment by medical vs. psychiatric team	Not reported. Assessment during following year.	Attempters & Completers	attempts for medical team, 13% repeat attempts for psychiatrist. 0% suicide for medical team, 0.4% for psychiatrist.
Gibbons JS et al. 1978[30]	RCT / Psychiatric & Other	400	1 yr / 400	No / No	UK / NR	ED contact for deliberate self poisoning, not requiring immediate psychiatric treatment	Yes	Don't Know	Don't Know	Don't Know		Don't Know / Yes	No	No	Yes	Yes	Don't Know	Don't Know / Yes	Yes	Yes	social worker to assist with task oriented problem solving	Not reported. Assessment at one year.	Attempters	13.5 repeated self poisoning in treatment group & 14.5 in control 10%
Hawton K et al. 1981[31]	RCT / Psychiatric	96	1 yr / 96	No / No	UK / 25.2	Hospitalization for deliberate self poisoning	Yes	Yes	Yes	Yes	Yes / Yes / No		Yes / No	Yes / No	Yes	Yes	Don't Know / No	Yes	Yes	Yes	outpatient vs. home based therapy	Maximum of 3 months, 1st 2 as frequent as needed	Attempters & SI	repeated attempts in home-based, 15% in outpatients.

70

Evidence Table 2. RCT and CCTs Describing Suicide Interventions Continued

Author, Year	Study Design / Setting	Sample Size Enrolled	Follow Up Time Points / Follow Up	Veterans / Military	Country / Mean Age	Eligibility Criteria	Described as Randomized	Method of Randomization	Allocation Concealment	Similarity at Baseline between groups	Eligibility Criteria Specified	Outcome Assessor Blinded	Care provider blinded	Patients Blinded	Point estimates & measures of variability for primary outcomes variable	Randomized patients analyzed in group they were allocated to	Co-interventions avoided	Compliance acceptable	Drop-out rate described	Timing of Outcome Assessment Similar	Intervention	Duration of Treatment	Outcome	Adverse Events
Hawton K et al. 1987[32]	RCT / Psychiatric & Primary Care	80	9 mths / 65	No / No	UK / 29.3	Hospitalized for overdose, not in need of formal psychiatric care	Yes	Don't Know	Don't Know	Yes	Yes	Yes	No		Yes		Don't Know	Yes	Yes		brief problem oriented counseling	Not reported. Assessment at one year.	Attempters & Completers	1 patient in counseling group committed suicide, 15.4% in general practitioner group repeated, 7.3% in counseling repeated
Guthrie E et al. 2001[33]	RCT / Psychiatric	119	6 mths / 95	No / No	UK / 31.2	ED contact for deliberate self poisoning	Yes	Don't Know		Yes	Yes	Yes	No	Yes	Yes	Yes	Don't Know	Yes	Yes	Yes	four sessions of psychodynamic interpersonal therapy in patient's home	4 weekly at home sessions	Attempters & Completers & SI	9% repeated self-harm in intervention & 28% in control, no completers
Bennewith O et al. 2002[34]	RCT / Primary Care	1932	12 mths / 1932	No / No	UK / 32.6	Seen in ED for deliberate self harm	Yes	Don't Know	Don't Know	Yes	Yes	Yes	No	Yes	Yes	Yes	Don't Know	Don't Know	Yes	Yes	letter from GP, use of guidelines for GP to use	1 year after first self harm episode	Attempters	211 repeat self-harm in intervention group & 189 in the control
Clarke T et al. 2002[35]	RCT / Other	526	12 mths / 467	No / No	UK / 33	ED contact for deliberate self harm	Yes	Yes	Yes	Yes	Yes / Don't Know	No			Yes	Yes	Don't Know	Yes	Yes	Yes	case management led by nurse practitioner	1 year follow up after first admission	Attempters	19 readmitted in treatment & 25 in control

Evidence Table 2. RCT and CCTs Describing Suicide Interventions Continued

Author, Year	Study Design / Setting	Sample Size Enrolled	Follow Up Time Points / Follow Up	Veterans / Military	Country / Mean Age	Eligibility Criteria	Described as Randomized	Method of Randomization	Allocation Concealment	Similarity at Baseline between groups	Eligibility Criteria Specified	Outcome Assessor Blinded	Care provider blinded	Patients Blinded	Point estimates & measures of variability for primary outcomes variable	Randomized patients analyzed in group they were allocated to	Co-interventions avoided	Compliance acceptable	Drop-out rate described	Timing of Outcome Assessment Similar	Intervention	Duration of Treatment	Outcome	Adverse Events
Motto JA et al. 2001[37]	RCT / Psychiatric	843	1 yr/843 5 yrs/843 15 yrs/843	No / No	US / NR	Hospitalized for depression or suicidality	Yes	Don't Know	Don't Know		Yes	Don't Know		No	Yes		Don't Know	Don't Know	No		follow up letter	15 years from discharge	Completers	after 15 years there were 25 suicides in the contact group, & 26 in the no contact group.
Morgan HG et al. 1993[38]	RCT / Psychiatric	212	1 yr/212	No / No	UK / 30.1	Admission follow up episode of deliberate self harm	Yes	Yes	Don't Know		Yes	Don't Know		No	Yes		Yes	Don't Know	Don't Know	Yes	"green card" offering easy access to psychiatrist on call	1 year follow up after first admission	Attempters & Completers	No suicides occurred; 5 repeated self harm (serious threats) in experiment & 15 in control
Evans MO et al. 1999[39]	RCT / Other	827	6 mths/827	No / No	UK / 33.3	Hospitalization for deliberate self harm	Yes	Yes	Don't Know		Yes	Yes	No	No	Yes		Don't Know	Don't Know	Yes	Yes	"green card" offering 24 hr crisis phone consultation	6 months following discharge	Attempters	2 suicides in "green card" group & 1 in control
Carter GL et al. 2005[40]	RCT / Psychiatric	772	12 mths/772	No / No	Australia / NR	ED contact for deliberate self poisoning	Yes	Yes	Yes		Yes	Yes	NA	No	Yes		Don't Know	Yes	Yes	Yes	postcard sent at 1,2,3,4,6,8,10,12 months after discharge	12 months	Attempters	57 repeat self harm in intervention & 68 in control

72

Evidence Table 2. RCT and CCTs Describing Suicide Interventions Continued

Author, Year	Study Design / Setting	Sample Size Enrolled	Follow Up Time Points / Follow Up	Veterans / Military	Country / Mean Age	Eligibility Criteria	Described as Randomized	Method of Randomization	Allocation Concealment	Similarity at Baseline between groups	Eligibility Criteria Specified	Outcome Assessor Blinded	Care provider blinded	Patients Blinded	Point estimates & measures of variability for primary outcomes variable	Randomized patients analyzed in group they were allocated to	Co-interventions avoided	Compliance acceptable	Drop-out rate described	Timing of Outcome Assessment Similar	Intervention	Duration of Treatment	Outcome	Adverse Events
Waterhouse J et al. 1990[43]	RCT / Primary Care & Hospital	99	1 wk/ NR 16 wk/ NR	No / No	UK / NR	ED contact for para-suicidal act by self poisoning	Yes	Yes	Don't Know	Yes	Yes	No	No	No		Yes		Don't Know	Don't Know	Don't Know	hospitalization	16 months	Attempters & SI	at 16 weeks a total of 3 admitted & 4 discharged patients repeated parasuicide
Unutzer J et al. 2006[45]	RCT / Primary Care	1801	2 yrs/ NR	Yes / No	US / 71.2	Elderly with depression	Yes	Yes	Yes	Yes	No	Yes	Yes	No	Yes	Yes	Yes	Don't Know	Don't Know	Don't Know	collaborative care program, including a depression case manager in primary care clinic	12 months	Completers & SI	No completed suicides during 2 year follow up
Mishara BL et al. 2005[46]	CCT / Other	120	2 mths/ 120 6 mths/ 120	No / No	Canada / NR	Family friend (of suicidal men) who called suicide hotline	No	No	Don't Know	Don't Know	Yes	No	No	No	Yes	Don't Know	Don't Know	Yes	Yes	Yes	family friend of suicidal men were assigned to one of four programs	post test after 2 months with 6 month follow up	Attempters	22.0% attempt rate at entry, 10.6% at 2 mo, 2.7% at 6 mo.

Evidence Table 3. Studies Describing Interventions Restricting the Access to Firearms

Author, Year	Study Design	Country / Setting	Veteran / Military	Legislation	Study Period	Outcome	Results
Loftin C et al. 1991[47]	Interrupted Time Series	US / Population	No / No	District of Columbia's Firearms Control Regulations Act 1976	1968–1987	Mean number of suicides per month	Suicides using firearms decreased from 2.6 per month to 2.0 per month (p=.005). Non-firearm related suicides did not experience a decrease of similar magnitude.
Ludwig J et al. 2000[48]	Interrupted Time Series	US / Population	No / No	Brady Handgun Violence Prevention Act, 1994	1985–1997	Total suicide rates per 100,000 of population for adults (≥21 years and ≥55 years) controlling for age, race, poverty and income levels, urban residence, and alcohol consumption, the effected states (32 states where Brady handgun act was implemented)	Firearm suicide rates declined by 0.32 (95% CI: -0.73, 0.20) for adults over 21 years old. For adults 55 or older suicide rates declined by 0.92 (95% CI: -1.43, -0.42, p<.05).
Lott JR et al. 2001[49]	Interrupted Time Series	US / Population	No / No	State Safe-Storage laws passed between October 1, 1989 through January 1, 1996	1979–1996	Comparison of suicide rates, accidental deaths and crimes in states with and without Safe-Storage laws	Regression estimates were not statistically significant from 0 or from each other with and without including control variables. Thus the gun laws did not seem to have a statistically significant effect on suicide rates.
Rosengart M et al. 2005[50]	Interrupted Time Series	US / Population	No / No	Multi-State: "Shall issue" (concealed weapons), minimum age of private purchase 21, minimum age of private possession 21, Junk gun per month, Junk gun ban	1979–1998	A cross sectional time series study of firearm suicides and homicides	None of the 5 laws were associated with a statistically significant change in firearm suicide rates. Of the 63,954 suicides between 1976-2001, 62% were committed with firearms. Firearm suicides increased from 2.6 in 1976 to a high of 5.7 in 1994. They quickly decreased to 2.5 in 2001. For youth between 14-17 child access prevention laws at the state level are associated with a 10.8% decrease in firearm suicides (RR, 0.89; 95% CI: 0.83-0.96). For adults between 18-20 state child access prevention laws are associated with a 11.1% decrease in suicides from firearms (RR, 0.89; 95% CI: 0.85-0.93).
Webster et al. 2004[51]	Interrupted Time Series	US / Population	No / No	State and federal Child Access Prevention laws (requiring safe storage)	1976–2001	Number of total suicides per 100,000 and methods used for youth between 14 to 20 years old	The mean percent of suicides by firearms decreased significantly after the legislation went into effect (23.2% to 16.2%, difference 7%, p<0.0001). The total number of suicides did not significantly decrease.
Rich CL et al. 1990[52]	Interrupted Time Series	Canada & US / Population	No / No	1978 Criminal Code of Canada	1973–1983	Number of suicides in Ontario and Toronto and method of suicide for Toronto	The suicide rate did not change significantly from the 5 years before and the 5 years after the 1978 gun control law (13.5 to 12.8, p=0.12). Regression analysis found no slope for the 5 years following the legislation.
Carrington PJ et al. 1994[53]	Interrupted Time Series	Canada / Population	No / No	1978 Criminal Code of Canada	1965–1977	Mean suicide rates per 100,000 and trends.	Suicide by firearm rates decreased after Bill C-51 (4.27 to 2.09, p=0.05). But the total suicide rate increased, suggesting that people turned to other methods.
Lester D et al. 1993[54]	Interrupted Time Series	Canada / Population	No / No	Canada's Criminal Law Amendment Act of 1977 (Bill C-51)	1969–1985	Annual suicide rates per 100,000 by all methods.	Before the passage of Bill C-51, firearm suicide rate was increasing (simple linear regression slope, b= 0.608, p=0.01), as were the total suicide rate and suicide rate from other methods. From 1978 to 1985 the overall suicide rate did not change and the rate by other methods did not change. The percentage of suicides by firearms did decrease (b= -0.574, p=0.03).
Lester D et al. 1994[55]	Interrupted Time Series	Canada & US / Population	No / No	Comment on assertion that Bill C-51 did not lessen suicide rates	1969–1991	Change in suicide rates for the period following the 1977 Bill C-51.	

74

Evidence Table 3. Studies Describing Interventions Restricting the Access to Firearms, Continued

Author, Year	Study Design	Country / Setting	Veteran / Military	Legislation	Study Period	Outcome	Results
Leenaars AA et al. 1996[56]	Interrupted Time Series	Canada / Population	No / No	Canada's Criminal Law Amendment Act of 1977 (Bill C-51)	1969-1985	Suicide rates before (1969-1976) and after (1978-1985) the enactment of Bill C-51	Suicide rates by firearms decreased significantly (p<0.05) after the passage of Bill C-51. Also the percentage of suicides by firearms also significantly decreased.
Lester D et al. 2001[57]	Interrupted Time Series	Canada / Population	No / No	Canada's Criminal Law Amendment Act of 1977 (Bill C-51)	1970-1995	Firearm suicide and homicide rates per 100,000	The correlation between year and the percentage of suicides and homicides by firearms is -0.86 (one-tailed p<0.001).
Leenaars AA et al. 1997[58]	Observational	Canada / Population	No / No	Canada's Criminal Law Amendment Act of 1977 (Bill C-51)	1969-1985	Suicide and homicide rates per 100,000 before and after Bill C-51 was passed	The mean annual number suicides decreased for those in the following age groups 15-24 (p<0.001), 35-64 (p<0.05), and 75 and over (p<0.01). Prior to the law the rate of suicides was increasing (regression line slope = 0.16) where as after the law went into effect the rate began to decrease (regression line slope = -0.13)
Leenaars AA et al. 2003[59]	Interrupted Time Series	Canada / Population	No / No	Canada's Criminal Law Amendment Act of 1977 (Bill C-51)	1969-1985	Suicide rates compared from before and after the 1977 Bill C-51.	Least squares regression showed that the introduction of the Bill had no statistically significant increase or decrease in the rate of suicides, overall or by firearms. However the Bill had a negative effect on the slope of the line, thus the Bill decreased the trend in suicide rates.
Bridges FS 2004[60]	Interrupted Time Series	Canada / Population	No / No	Canadian Bill C-17		Total suicide and homicide rates per 100,000, as well as methods, before and after Bill C-17.	The mean annual number of suicides significantly decreased from the first 7 year period to the 7 years following instatement of the Bill (4.09 to 3.17, p=.001). The rates by other methods increased significantly (9.02 to 9.76, p=.01). The total average number of suicides did not significantly differ between the 2 study periods (13.11 to 12.93).
Chung AH et al 2005[61]	Interrupted Time Series	Canada / Population	No / No	Canadian Bill C-17	1984-1998	Suicide rates and methods for youth between the ages of 15-19 before and after Bill C-17.	The percent of suicide by firearms decreased from 55% in 1979 to 25% in 1999. Death by other means increased during this time. The overall rate of suicides did not decrease.
Snowdon J et al. 1992[62]	Observational	Australia / Population	No / No	Several?	1979-1999	Suicide rates per 100,000 by gender, State, age and residence.	The mean rate of firearm suicides was 6.13 for men and 0.43 for women (p<0.005).
Chapman S et al 2006[63]	Interrupted Time Series	Australia / Population	No / No	1996 gun law reform, following the 1996 firearm massacre in Tasmania	1968-1989	Changes in trends of total firearm suicides and suicides per 100,000 of population.	Before 1996, annual average of 491.7 firearm suicides. From 1997 to 2003, annual average of 246.6 firearm suicides.
Cantor CH et al. 1995[64]	Observational	Australia / Population	No / No	Weapons Act 1990 (Qld)	1979-2003	Firearm suicide mean annual rates per 100,000 and method for different geographical areas two years before and two years after the legislation went into effect	Suicide rates decreased in metropolitan (3.6 to 2.3) and provincial areas (5.2 to 3.1) (p<0.05). The mean annual rate per 100,000 for rural areas was about double that of metropolitan and provincial areas. This rate did not decrease after the legislation. There was also a significant decrease in suicide rates among men and adults between 15 and 29 years old.
Ozanne-Smith J et al 2004[65]	Interrupted Time Series	Australia / Population	No / No	Victoria Response (1988) and Firearms Act of 1996	1990-1993	Following gun control regulations, death rates, trends, and ownership in Victoria and Australia.	The overall death rate decreased for Australia (-3.9%; 95% CI: -4.8% ro -3.1%) and Victoria(-4.9% 95% CI: -5.9, -3.9) from 1979 - 2000. Significant decreases in firearm related suicides were seen in Victoria. Suicides by firearms dropped by 54.5% from 1979 to 2000.
Beautrais A et al. 2006[66]	Interrupted Time Series	New Zealand / Population	No / No	Amendment to the Arms Act, 1992	1985-2002	Age-specific suicide rates per 100,000 of population for firearm and Non-firearm related suicides	For youths (15-24years), firearm suicides were reduced by 39% in the 3 year implementation period and decreased 66% in the 5 year post-implementation period. For adults (25+ years) firearm suicides decreased by 25% in the 3 year implementation period and decreased by 39% in the 5 year post-implementation period

75

APPENDIX D. PEER REVIEW COMMENTS

Appendix D. Peer Review Comments

Section	Comment	Change
General	Outcome information was collected for only three categories: "Attempters, Completers, SI." The synthesis project does not address any literature demonstrating if suicide prevention strategies impact: a) the need for hospitalization, b) number of ER visits, c) patient and provider satisfaction, etc.	The scope of the report was set in consultation with the ESP Advisory Committee and the outcomes were restricted to the ones included in this report. These additional outcomes could be included in an update or new ESP report
General	The literature review was detailed but narrative, and it would be helpful to see the summation in a data table. It's very difficult to find the "take home messages" amidst all the detail. There apparently were data collection forms in Appendix D. Would like to see data tables for the data collected in these forms to better understand the results of the synthesis project.	Summarizing the results of disparate studies is always a challenge. We have included Evidence Tables summarizing most of the data from the included studies in Appendix C. Each report section then also has a narrative summary, as does the report's conclusion.
General	Are there any studies on suicide prevention related to this report that we have overlooked?: The use of telemedicine for suicide prevention	We reported all studies identified as of the search date. We found no studies reporting outcomes from telemedicine interventions.
General	The VA National Center for Suicide Prevention and the MIRECC in Denver may have at least some published data describing the impact of the recent VA national suicide prevention hotline. This would obviously be the most relevant information, yet there was no mention of this in the project synthesis. It would be helpful if the document states explicitly one way or another if there is any recent data to be factored from either of these VA suicide prevention centers, either in the literature, in press or otherwise.	We used standard search techniques to find published literature, and did not attempt to identify unpublished or not yet published results. *We'll check with VA to see if there is anything published abpout the impact of the VA hotline.*
Executive Summary, Methods	even in this brief summary, it would be useful to list the inclusion criteria yielding studies below, e.g., interventions, controlled studies, outcomes limited to attempts, completed suicides?))	We have added a list of the search criteria in the executive summary.
Introduction, Background	Section contains much useful information; some statements would benefit from references, to guide the interested reader— e.g., what is known or theorized about media-induced imitation or contagion?	We have added a reference to a recent review on media-induced imitation.
Methods, Study Selection	This exclusion makes sense but doesn't seem to be consistently followed. I'll note examples below. If interional, maybe further clarification of the exclusion here would be useful	Our original description in Study Selection was imprecise. We have added text to clarify the search criteria, especially with respect to exclusion of mental health interventions.

Appendix D. Peer Review Comments Continued

Methods, Grade	I may have missed it, but it's not clear to me where these quantitative instructions are applied to the studies in this report. If in an appendix, might be useful to steer the reader to it here.	The quality assessment of individual articles appears in tables in Appendix C. The GRADE ratings were applied to sets of evidence taken together, and appear in the text of the results section.
Key Questions 1 & 2	All of these studies are quite well described. This one, though, left me with a question. Did the study employ a chaplain to deliver a secular counseling/educational intervention? Or was there a religious component to the education? Seems basic to understanding the study/	The article in question does not provide enough detail to allow us to accurately answer this question.
Key Questions 1 & 2	Referring to Koons et al. This study would seem to be excluded as a "mental health intervention only". Its foundational efficacy studies specifically addressed suicide. If there's a reason to include it, consider clarifying criteria?	See answer to item 8
Key Questions 1 & 2	referring to Ilgen Also would seem to be excluded as a "mental health intervention only". If SUD or 'program' features set it apart, consider clarifying criteria?	See answer to item 8
Key Questions 1 & 2	referring to Gibbons Would seem to be excluded as a "mental health intervention only". If reason is that the study addresses an induction effect rather than a treatment effect, consider clarifying here.	See answer to item 8
Key Questions 1 & 2	referring to Webster et al. Not sure I understand, because it's not clear to me how representative any one state is (of the country?) Consider listing states and characteristics, e.g., more rural, higher prevalence of alcoholism, etc.?	We have re-written the description of this study's results to avoid the question of "representativeness."
Limitations, Study Quality	I'm sure the authors know more about this than I do; I thought this work consistutes a 'systematic review' and that a 'meta-analysis' would be distinguished from this review by the pooling of data across studies.	This comment is correct, this synthesis is not a meta-analysis and we have changed the text to reflect that.
Executive Summary, Key Questions 1 & 2	What about access to and treatment of mental health or sud disorders– does that reduce suicide – addiction treatment, clozapine, etc	See answer to item 8
Executive Summary, Key Question 3	Perhaps a major statement here on defining terms is needed – this is really a problem in the literature. Define gesture, attempt, ideation, death ideation etc.	We have added more text highlighting the critical nature of such terminology for advancing the field.

Appendix D. Peer Review Comments Continued

Section	Comment	Response
Methods, Figure 1	Alcohol and drug use isn't listed as a factor involved in behavior – this seems like an oversight	We have added a comment about the role of substance abuse and other factors not explicitly appearing in the Mann conceptual model to the introduction.
	Another target might be social situation – homelessness, employment (there is a strong correlation in the jobless rate and suicide rates) so programs like CWT or Supported employment might be important to mention.	Same answer as item 18.
Methods	How about those in mh care	See answer to item 8
Methods	Transition from inpatient to outpatient care – I believe there is data on a critical time intervention by lisa dixon on this issue	We found no study by Dixon reporting a direct effect on suicide attempts or completions.
Methods	It isn't clear what this means: " were rejected at title review as clearly irrelevant to the project"	If the title clearly indicated that the study did not report an outcome relevant to our search, then it was rejected. This is standard practice in systematic reviews and meta-analyses.
Results, Literature Flow	The prospect study (M Bruce showed a reduction in suicide ideation when treating depression in primary care, should these type studys not be included?	We did not consider studies reporting changes in rates of suicidal ideation, only studies that reported direct effects on suicide attempts or completions.
Key Questions 1 & 2	Probably worth saying in the summary: "Our review did not focus on purely menthal health interventions. These have been the subject of other reviews. Perhaps somewhat surprisingly given the role of depressive disorders as significant risk factors for suicide, the evidence in support of the use of antidepressants is rather weak"	See answer to item 8
Limitations	However, I am at a loss to explain why the IMPACT study was discussed but the PROSPECT study was excluded given the extremely similar study designs (perhaps because IMPACT included some VA sites?).	If the study reported including veterans, then it was included, but not otherwise. See item 8.
General	This manuscript is still at a developmental stage so I delineate that which I would like to see in a final version more than providing a peer review per se [interspersed with other editorial observations roughly in order of appearance]:	No reply needed.
General	An initial discussion of known correlates of suicide and suicidality (manuscript leads off suggesting the primary one is substance abuse) and/or conceptual framework for approaching this topic	In the Introduction, we described the Mann review's conceptual model in moderate detail, because we used its search strategy. Our goal was not to review existing conceptual frameworks or to develop new ones.
Introduction		

Appendix D. Peer Review Comments Continued

	Greater connection and discussion to policy issues and programs; at present it is a very dry list of vignettes from research papers	The results section lists in a narrative format the results of our search. The summary section contains some comments related to research and policy development.
Results Key Question 1	Summary of strategies for key question #1 is largely absent	Questions 1 and 2 were answered together.
Results	Specific data from the quality review are not presented	The quality data appear in Appendix C for the RCTs and CCTs.
General	Page numbers end partway into the manuscript	This problem has been fixed.
General	Needs editing for consistency of tone and some substitution of colloquial or inappropriate word choices [e.g., 'repertoire', 'more easily had']	These phrases have been rewritten.
Executive Summary, Key Question 3	Page 10, penultimate paragraph: would revise to "similar…profiles to the antemortem profiles of suicide completers."	We have made the suggested change.
Introduction	Page 14, first paragraph: consider "nonclinician gatekeepers," such as "medical clerks, chaplains, or military unit commanders," since education programs may provide gatekeeper education to staff at medical facilities	We have made the suggested change.
Introduction	Page 14, last paragraph: brief summaries miss some elements (firearm purchase background checks and waiting periods; drug package configurations not just sizes)	We have made the suggested change.
General	Beautrais study: should describe the nature of the additional data; as it reads now it is not clear what distinction is being made in the last sentence	We have added a brief description of the additional data to clarify this point.
General	The objectives of the report are not clear. Why was this report commissioned? In response to what pressures? Several key questions were developed following a conference call (page 14). It is not clear who commissioned the Office of R&D for the Evidence Synthesis Project; why were these topics (i.e suicide screening) selected. What were the "key questions" responding to? Why was a key question formulated but not addressed at all in the review?? Therefore, in my opinion additional background might be helpful to better delineate whether the objectives and scope of the report were appropriate. On the other hand, the methods are clearly described.	As noted in the report, this topic was nominated by Office of Research and Development to the ESP Advisory Committee, and the Key Questions were developed by these two groups working together. The pressures leading to the nomination of this topic, other than VA's concern for the mental health of the veteran population, are outside our scope.

79

Appendix D. Peer Review Comments Continued

General	I was impressed with the objectivity of the report. Studies are presented without bias. The strengths and weaknesses of the studies are briefly but clearly described. After each topic, the results of the relevant studies pertaining to that topic are summarized. These are strengths of the review.	No changes needed.
General	Are there any studies on suicide prevention related to this report that we have overlooked?: No to my knowledge. Critical studies that have influenced national VHA policy regarding suicide screening and intervention have been included. One possible criticism is that studies that have been pivotal should be identified as such and perhaps discussed more fully. An example might be the US Air Force Study from the BMJ (Knox et al, reference #14).	We agree the methodological advantages of the Knox study and have added extra detail about it.
General	This report is well constructed, well written and very helpful. It summarizes a broad range of studies, providing brief commentary in the form of summary statements. The report stops short of suggesting national guidelines or policy based upon the available data (i.e. evidence based recommendations), potentially a limitation as the authors are probably particularly well poised to do so after this thorough review. In fact, Key Question #1 directly asks this question and is left unanswered. The responses to Key Questions #1 and #2 are tentative and very general. For example, the response to Key Question #3 suggests that preliminary data be collected from the computerized medical record (page 8), without discussing any specific thoughts or recommendations as to what data should be collected and how. The use of the computer to help address Key Question #2 is not mentioned although the ability to track patients and ensure that they receive appropriate interventions is a very well recognized use of this resource.	The purpose of the report was to conduct a literature review, not report a policy analysis. We included a few general recommendations in the conclusion. Key Questions 1 and 2 were answered together.
Key Questions 1, 2, & 3		
Executive Summary	Page 8 suggest choosing another word than "Rare" in first sentence. Current debate in Congress, press, and email is why rates are so high for veterans. It might be the wrong tone to set.	We have removed that word and simplified the statement.

Appendix D. Peer Review Comments Continued

General	Are there any studies on suicide prevention related to this report that we have overlooked?: Is there any work from VISN19 MIRECC which was designed to focus on suicide issues that might assist with this analysis?	We used standard search techniques to find published literature. *We'll check with the MIRECC to see if there is anything additional we might have missed.*
General	This review demonstrated an embarrassing lack of evidence for Veterans in this critical and highly publicized topic. Research $$ should be directed toward remedying this. Perhaps a combination of the currently funded VISN 19 MIRECC and new studies?	No changes needed.
General	After reading this review and the synthesis review on depression, there seems a consistent theme in those studies having positive impact of additional or directed staff who build a "relationship" with the patient that plays the role of support and intervention as well as providing social contact for discussion, venting of issues, and advice. Perhaps the social isolation component should be studied as a variable that might have predictive value?	We agree that such factors are likely to be important. We have added a comment about this in the conclusion.
General	Consider studies involving telebuddy type devices, web access and response, etc.	No studies of such interventions were identified.

www.ingramcontent.com/pod-product-compliance
Lightning Source LLC
Chambersburg PA
CBHW081555170526
45166CB00009B/2709